AIDS:

WHAT THE DISCOVERERS OF HIV HAVE NEVER ADMITTED

LATEST EDITION

LAWRENCE BROXMEYER MD

© 2014 Lawrence Broxmeyer MD
All Rights Reserved
Registered: US Library of Congress

ISBN: 1495457044
ISBN 13: 9781495457043

TABLE OF CONTENTS

PROLOGUE v

INTRODUCTION 1

1. EPIDEMIC 21

2. CATS 27

3. CANCER STRUGGLES 33

4. SHYH-CHING LO 41

5. IN THE SEMEN OF MAN 49

6. THE TRAGIC COST OF PREMATURE CONSENSUS 69

7. THE RACE 73

8. SMOKE AND MIRRORS 81

9. FABRICATED SLAUGHTER 89

10. VIRAL DELUSIONS 101

11. LUCKY 107

PROLOGUE

In *HIV Equals AIDS and Other Myths of the AIDS War*, Dr. Gary Null's summary is well taken: "Since 1984 the mainstream media have been giving us only one side of the AIDS story—the officially approved side. When Dr. Robert Gallo and then Secretary of Health Margaret Heckler announced that the probable cause of AIDS had been discovered, HIV became the sole cause of AIDS, and the case was closed."

"Overnight, the word 'probable' ceased to exist and it became dogma ... engraved in stone," adds investigative journalist John Lauritsen. From that time on, a campaign has been conducted to program us into believing that the human immunodeficiency virus is a deadly, infectious virus that inevitably results in AIDS, and death. And we have been continually told that while no cure exists, antiviral drugs, including AZT, DDI, and DDC, will slow down the progression of the disease. Despite evidence to the contrary, the general public continues to buy these ideas. They are the only ones reported. The fact is, there have always been people questioning or disagreeing with the official theory and treatment approach, but they have been silenced. Early on, the theory was challenged by a world-renowned retrovirologist, Peter Duesberg, professor of biochemistry and molecular biology at the University of California at Berkeley, and by Nobel Prize-winning scientist Walter Gilbert. But instead of being urged on in their attempt to help mankind, they were ridiculed and their funding was stopped."

Indeed, few people in the world know more about retroviruses than Dr. Peter Duesberg, who was one of the pioneers in defining their ultrastructure. And in his book *Inventing the AIDS Virus*, he asserts that HIV, like virtually all retroviruses, is harmless. Duesberg also mentions that HIV meets none of the usual criteria (such as the six laws of virology) used to establish that a microbe causes disease. But if that is so, why do scientists persist in saying that AIDS is an epidemic caused by HIV? As Duesberg tells it, the federal Centers for Disease Control and Prevention needed a serious epidemic to justify its continued existence, and by naming AIDS a single contagious disease, it created an atmosphere of public fear that brought it increased funding and power. The biomedical establishment took note. Having failed to find a viral cause of cancer, Duesberg says, virus hunters needed a new disease, and AIDS was it. The HIV-AIDS connection was then announced by Robert Gallo, head of a retrovirus lab at the National Cancer Institute, at a 1984 press conference rather than demonstrated in a peer-reviewed scientific paper. Further, Duesberg mentions, the pharmaceutical companies exploited the situation by bringing back highly toxic failed cancer drugs, such as AZT, which, he says, destroys the immune system and causes AIDS-like symptoms. Duesberg also cites other scientists who have questioned the HIV-AIDS hypothesis, among them several Nobel laureates, including Kary Mullis (for chemistry), who wrote the foreword for *Inventing the AIDS Virus*.

INTRODUCTION

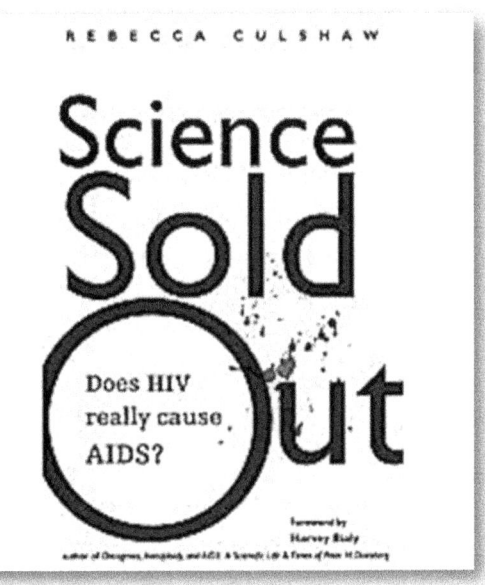

Once upon a time, a small group of politically powerful scientists rammed a flawed theory of the origin and cause of AIDS down America's and then the world's throat.

Yet we are still led to believe that we are fortunate, even 'lucky' that retroviruses, only discovered in the 1970s, were uncovered just in time to label them the culprit in a killer AIDS epidemic. And 'lucky' that two "HIVs" were discovered in rapid succession, and the technology and theory to link AIDS to the "HIV" retrovirus were fully in place for the first time in history, only a few years prior to the recognition of the AIDS epidemic.

Lucky? The latest statistics released as of this writing by the Centers for Disease Control and Prevention, which still labels AIDS an "epidemic," say otherwise:

> "CDC estimates that 1,144,500 persons aged 13 years and older [in the United States] are living with HIV infection, including 180,900 (15.8%) who are unaware of their infection.[1] Over the past decade, the number of people living with HIV has increased, while the annual number of new HIV infections has remained relatively stable. Still, the pace of new infections continues at far too high a level..."[1]

In other words, with regard to AIDS, over the last decade we have been going nowhere, fast.

And, as if further proof was needed, according to the National Institute of Allergy and Infectious Diseases (NIAID), despite the global public health community's best efforts to prevent new infections, 2.6 million people around the world became newly infected with HIV in 2009 alone. And although most do not have access to antiretroviral HIV drugs, many (approximately 5 million people) did, with the following results.

> "A growing proportion of patients receiving long-term antiretroviral therapy are experiencing treatment failure, drug toxicities, side effects, and drug resistance. In this regard, recent studies have noted an increased incidence of malignancies, cardiovascular and metabolic complications, and premature aging associated with long-term HIV disease or antiretroviral therapy."

http://www.niaid.nih.gov/news/newsreleases/2011/Pages/ AIDSat30.aspx

When the 20th anniversary of the first reported AIDS cases passed, AIDS had infected nearly 60 million people around the world, of which almost 22 million, including nearly half a million Americans, had died, and 8,500 AIDS deaths occurred daily. Yet the prospects for a cure or vaccine are as remote as they were three decades ago.

Obviously a reassessment of what we are doing wrong with regard to our present thoughts about and treatment of "HIV/AIDS" is badly needed, and according to one website, almost 3,000 scientists, doctors, and educators have expressed doubts about the makeshift, contrived evidence provided to this point that "HIV" causes AIDS. And they include several Noble laureates.
http://www.rethinkingaids.com/quotes/rethinkers.htm

Nevertheless, the mantra that "HIV is the sole cause of AIDS" is so well known and accepted universally that any suggestion to the contrary is usually met with disdain by the AIDS establishment. One notable example of this disdain was provided by Taiwanese-born *TIME* magazine's Man of the Year in 1996, AIDS researcher David Da-i Ho, MD, who famously and absurdly declared, "It's the virus, stupid!"[2]

Despite such blather, it is important to realize that the statement "HIV is the sole cause of AIDS" is still just a hypothesis. There are unanswered questions and controversy concerning the role of HIV as the sole cause of AIDS, let alone the cause of AIDS at all. And until they are resolved, a cure is not possible.

First, let me say that, having treated AIDS patients and having done AIDS-based research during and after the deadly US AIDS coastal epidemic—with peer-reviewed studies to that effect including one published in the *Journal of Infectious Diseases*—it is inconceivable to me that anyone can address the question of AIDS origin without seeing that it began as a highly transmittable infectious disease that could be sexually transmitted.

Let me assure you, to think differently is merely to box oneself into a scientifically untenable position. The case of Gaëtan Dugas alone, the French Canadian Air Canada flight attendant who single-handedly infected—either by himself or by passing it to his sexual contacts—40 new cases of AIDS, speaks differently, much differently.

On the other hand, the growing number of scientists, virologists among them, who doubt that the HIV retrovirus, or any other retrovirus, could be behind the AIDS epidemic, stand on firm ground.

So firm, in fact, that eventually Dr. Luc Montagnier himself, HIV's primary discoverer, came out with his "cofactor" theory, which basically admitted that HIV in and of itself could not even approach the destruction rendered in AIDS patients.

So the emphasis here—and I might add, the only correct emphasis—will not be on whether AIDS can be caused by an infectious factor, but on whether the so-called human immunodeficiency virus is really a virus or retrovirus to begin with.

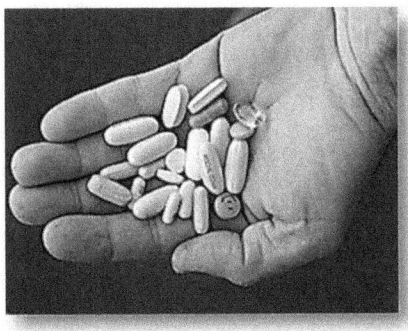

Figure 1. One HIV Regimen, Supposedly "Antiretroviral," Like the Pills in This Patient's Hand, Seemingly Keeps "AIDS" at Bay but Can Take a Harsh Physical Toll.

One argument often used by HIV pharmaceutical-sponsored devotees is to show how their antiretrovirals increase life-spans of AIDS victims. But does highly active antiretroviral therapy (HAART) really prolong lives? Depends on how you look at it. To some orthodox believers, yes, by an average of 13–15 years, and there are studies, many of which are pharmaceutically sponsored, to show this. But to others, this is absurd—citing that the rate of death among "HIV/AIDS patients" was just being increasingly redefined and manipulated by the HIV powers that be to include illnesses less life-threatening than those behind the original AIDS epidemic.

Yet, though HAART might or might not greatly prolong life on the average, there is at least some reliable testimony that individuals have experienced clinical improvement on it, often dramatic and immediate. However, logic insists that such immediate benefit cannot be the result of any antiretroviral action whose supposed benefits (decrease in 'viral load', rise in CD4) come slowly. Rather, such testimony likely reflects an antibiotic or anti-inflammatory effect.

If such antiretrovirals are indeed exerting an antibiotic affect, the question then becomes: Which microorganism (and not virus) are they hitting? Kirk et al. reported that antiretrovirals cause a marked decrease in the incidence of TB, and to an even larger extent, fowl tuberculosis (*Mycobacterium avium*), which many experts consider inevitable with AIDS.[3] And unlike what the manufacturers of such antiretrovirals would like to hear, Kirk was hard pressed to ascribe the significantly lower risk of fowl tuberculosis in AIDS to merely an increased CD4 immune cell count as a result of antiretrovirals. Rather, such a dramatic drop in tubercular *Mycobacterial avium* suggested to Kirk a direct effect on the part of "antiretrovirals" against AIDS-borne fowl tuberculosis.

This opens up the interesting question of whether "antiretrovirals" aren't acting more like poorly designed, super-expensive, antitubercular agents and increasing CD4 counts merely by suppressing typical and atypical forms of TB. It has always been terribly important to pharmaceutical interests to give the impression to both the lay and scientific communities that their "antiretrovirals", and only their "antiretrovirals", could increase a CD4 immune count in the blood of AIDS patients. Yet we know that one of the most dramatic restorations of CD4 count on record occurred in patients with "HIV" and TB, when only anti-TB treatment was used—as in John's study where a CD4 count of 89/ll climbed to 760/ll.[4] This of course doesn't fit into Big Pharma's agenda, since all anti-TB antibiotics are now off patent and cannot generate nearly the profit of their antiretroviral counterparts.

Just as disconcerting to American pharmaceutical interests was the unexpected finding in early AIDS autopsies of the surprisingly high proportion of difficult-to-diagnose fowl tuberculosis,[5] or *Mycobacterium avium-intracellulare*, in up to 55% of American cases in early studies.[6] Actually, in all likelihood this American percentage was much higher, as statistics used did not include respiratory and gastrointestinal colonization without clinically evident infection. According to the NIAID, TB is still the major attributable cause of death in AIDS patients.

Pharmaceutical interests could not just ignore this, so they began publishing studies that showed how with antiretrovirals tubercular infection dramatically declined (see figure 2).[6] Even the NIH's ears perked up, and they began funding grants to better ascertain just why HIV antiretrovirals mysteriously suppressed atypical and typical forms of tuberculosis.

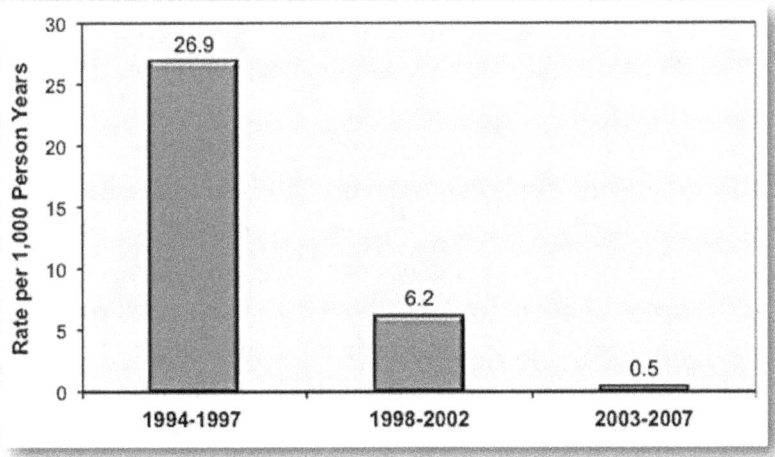

Figure 2. Incidence of Disseminated Fowl Tuberculosis (*Mycobacterium avium complex*) Infections in US AIDS. The HIV Outpatient Study 1994–2007. Figure is based on data from Buchacz K, Baker RK, Patella FJ Jr, et al. AIDS-defining opportunistic illnesses in US patients, 1994–2007: a cohort study. *AIDS*, 2010; 24:1549–59.

Then there was the purposeful loosening of criteria by HIV scientists to include tuberculosis—which infects, according to the CDC, a third of the world—and fowl tuberculosis as "AIDS-defining" illnesses, a move that was no more and no less than simply a survival strategy to keep the HIV hypothesis viable. HIV diehards realized early that up to 70% of people with TB were "HIV-positive". And although there were other "AIDS-defining" illnesses postulated, none came close to the number of people infected with TB. Besides, early HIV investigators knew very well that not only were tubercular mycobacterial infections the main cause of bacterial infection in AIDS, but they often preceded other infections in AIDS by one to ten months.[8]

So above all, tuberculosis had to be made an "AIDS-defining" illness. In fact, the definition of HIV now, thanks to the industry's active efforts, has become so loosely constructed that even patients with verifiable tuberculosis and no HIV, who nonetheless reacted positively for HIV, can be included under the umbrella of having AIDS, despite the fact that they admittedly do not have HIV.

Nowhere were the hypersensitivity and evasive tactics of such "HIV experts" on display toward tuberculosis and its related mycobacteria than in the 2005 book titled *Retroviral Testing and Quality Assurance Essentials for Laboratory Diagnosis.*[9] Here, forgetful HIV "experts" left out (on page 24) TB and its related mycobacteria from their list of medical conditions suspected or known to produce false-positive screening and western blot tests in AIDS. Included among these experts were those from the University of Maryland's Laboratory of Viral Diagnostics, the Institute of Human Virology, the FDA, the Director of the National Serology Reference Laboratory in Australia, the World Health Organization (WHO) and the Centre on HIV/AIDS (also in Australia). And the fact that this entire group studiously ignored what is hands down the biggest cause of such AIDS false-positive screening tests and "indeterminate" Western blots didn't even seem to faze them. Moreover, that this was oversight on the part of these HIV experts is extremely doubtful if one knows the history involved.

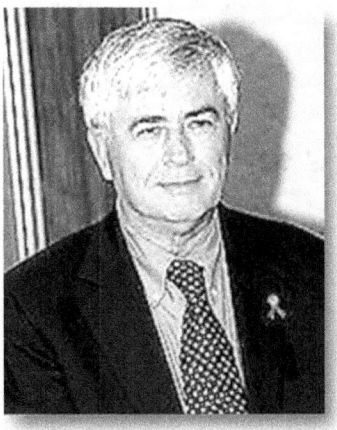

Figure 3. Veterinarian Max Myron Essex, a Key Figure in Early "HIV" Research.

Well known as the first scientist to propose HIV testing, veterinarian Max Myron Essex knew that tuberculosis gives a false positive for "HIV" in almost 70% of cases. In fact such cross-reactivity between HIV and tubercular pathogens was so significant, that it forced Essex and his protégé, Oscar Kashala, to warn that both the HIV screening test, the enzyme-linked immunosorbent assay (ELISA) and western blot results "should be interpreted with caution when screening individuals with *M. tuberculosis* or other mycobacterial species."[10] This, of course, automatically meant throwing away HIV serum diagnostics for at least a third of the people in the known world—and that fraction doesn't even include those who harbor *M. avium*, the fowl tuberculosis so common in AIDS as well.

Oscar Kashala graduated as an internist from the Kinshasa University Medical School in his native Congo, at a point when the AIDS epidemic was just beginning. He met Veterinarian Max Essex when Essex visited Africa to find out more about AIDS and how to further his ambitions to prove that it was caused by a retrovirus. Max offered Oscar a position in Boston as an AIDS research fellow, and for the next decade Kashala did clinical AIDS research for the US pharmaceutical industry.

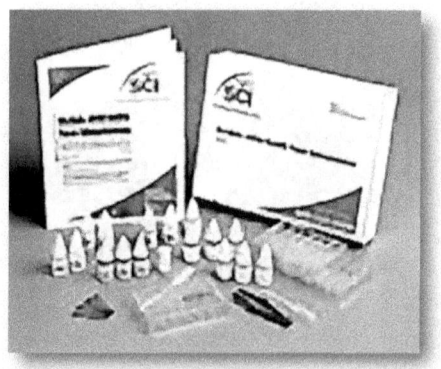

Figure 4. The ELISA "HIV/AIDS" Screening Test

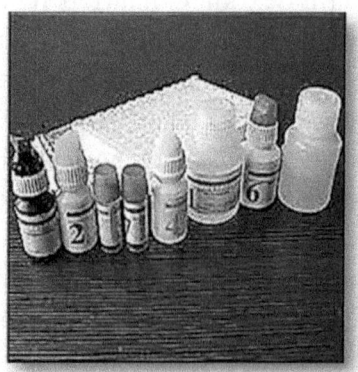

Figure 5. Western Blot Test to Confirm the Person Is "HIV-Positive."

There were other problems in the proclamation that AIDS antiretrovirals extended lives an average of 15 years, and they soon became apparent. While the original AIDS patients were desperately ill, many of them showing fowl tuberculosis early in their disease presumably through rectal transmission…as time went on, not all cases of "AIDS-defining" TB were ill, many of them being dormant or asymptomatic. Such "AIDS" individuals, of course, would survive longer. In the meantime, with all the literature saying that antiretrovirals increase the life of AIDS patients, with or without such drugs, the greatest risk of death from "HIV" disease remained 35–45 years old (median age), much as when AIDS began.

And then there was the terrible toxicity of these antiretrovirals. The fact that certain studies claim that antiretrovirals extend the life of an AIDS patient does not mean that they are benign in the least. As just one example, and putting aside the black-box warnings regarding liver failure, kidney failure, and severe neuropathy—many cardiac complications of "HIV" are not affected by antiretroviral cocktails (HAART) and such heart problems continue to develop in AIDS, either with antiretroviral treatment or because of antiretroviral treatment. This is because viral treatment itself can cause a metabolic syndrome, characterized by altered body-fat distribution and an insulin resistance. This, together with other factors that such retroviral cocktails create, is associated with increased atherosclerosis and subsequent risk of peripheral artery and coronary artery diseases such as heart attacks.[11]

Also, in the HIV-positive population of patients receiving highly active antiretroviral therapy (HAART), there has been an increase in the incidence of severe facial lipoatrophy (facial wasting), at times quite grotesque.

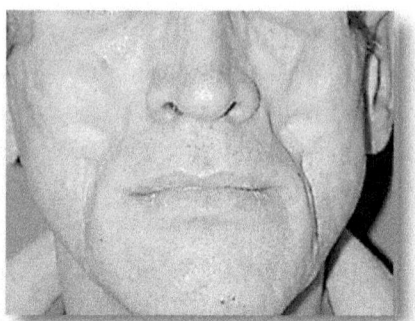

Figure 6. Facial Lipoatrophy from Antiretrovirals.

By 2000, French retrovirologist Luc Montagnier—at least the co-discoverer, and in the eyes of many, the discoverer of HIV—who seldom saw a retrovirus that he didn't feel was either infective or lethal to humans—said, "It is tuberculosis that constitutes the greatest public health problem today: 1.7 billion people have latent infections of *Mycobacterium tuberculosis* [the bacillus that causes tuberculosis], while eight million are actively infected."[12]

Actually, in 1990, tuberculosis killed more people than any other single disease—some estimate almost three million. Perhaps, then, it might have been better, therefore, had Montagnier synthesized such thoughts into his hypothesized retroviral cause of AIDS. For example:

The first reports of fowl tuberculosis in US AIDS appeared in 1982, the year previous to Montagnier and Barré-Sinoussi's original Pasteur report on their mysterious retrovirus. At UCLA, Zakowski[13] found that "All of the homosexual patients that have died of acquired immunodeficiency at the UCLA Medical Center for the Health Sciences have had disseminated MAC [fowl tuberculosis] infection." Furthermore, the team said, "Because of this preliminary observation, we now vigorously seek evidence of mycobacteria [tubercular] infection in homosexuals with unexplained lymphadenopathy [a disease or disorder of enlarged or inflamed lymph nodes]." Zakowski, in fact, mentions that he did not feel it unreasonable to treat AIDS patients empirically for fowl tuberculosis, pending the results of mycobacterial cultures, even if acid-fast [tubercular] bacilli are not identified on smears or tissue sections." In fact, in the eyes of Zakowski and his colleagues, such antitubercular treatment could very well be lifesaving.

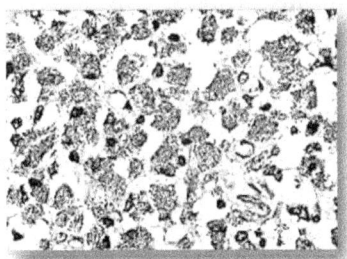

Figure 7. Mycobacterium avium (Fowl or Pig Tuberculosis) in the Lymph Node Tissue of an AIDS Victim. Ziehl-Neelsen Stain. Histopathology of lymph node above shows tremendous numbers of acid-fast tubercular bacilli in it. CDC/Dr. Edwin P. Ewing Jr.

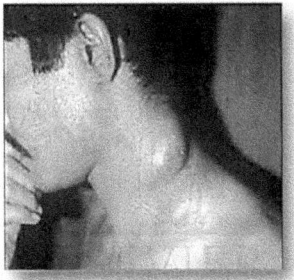

Figure 8. The Not-at-all Uncommon Tuberculosis of a Lymph Node [Lymphadenopathy] in the Neck.

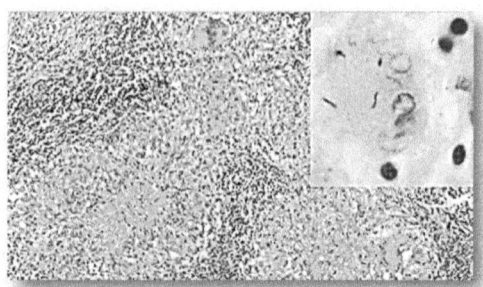

Figure 9. Microscopic Picture of TB of the Lymph Node. In the right upper corner insert are classical red tubercular acid-fast bacilli.

Both TB and fowl TB commonly affect human lymph nodes. Therefore, one can only wonder why Luc Montagnier not only ignored but didn't even consider the possibility of tuberculosis when sending Françoise Barré-Sinoussi in with his human HIV reverse-transcriptase Geiger counter to look exclusively for a "retrovirus" in their first gay victim with enlarged lymph nodes—a young man with large neck lymph nodes. After all, these first French AIDS specimens, taken in 1983, had a medically directed differential diagnosis protocol to follow, a list of other possibilities besides the retroviruses. In fact, soon thereafter McCabe appeared[14] in the *Journal of the American Medical Association* (*JAMA*), suggesting that not only did TB clearly predominate as the cause of enlarged lymph nodes in adults, but that atypical TB such as *Mycobacterium avium* (fowl TB) was hands down the number-one cause of infectious lymph node involvement in children. Shouldn't this have given Montagnier and Françoise Barré-Sinoussi pause and reason to test for such pathogens before attributing these first French AIDS lymph node specimens exclusively to a "retrovirus"? Apparently not, as not even the mention or afterthought of tuberculosis or fowl tuberculosis (*M. avium*) was in their report.

Yet despite this, it soon became obvious that TB and Fowl TB were the two leading causes of infectious death in AIDS, both having bacillary (a bacillus form) as well as viral forms—every bit as capable of throwing off signals for the reverse transcriptase registering on Montagnier and Françoise Barré-Sinoussi's equipment as retroviruses were.

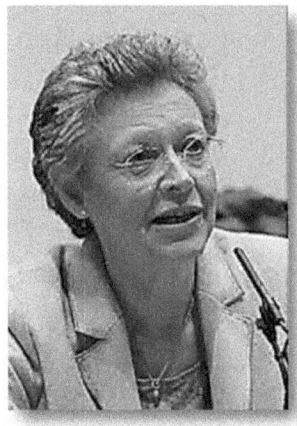

Figure 10. Virologist Françoise Barré-Sinoussi

From its first publication, "HIV" was questioned. Biochemist Kary Mullis, who in 1993 was ironically awarded the Nobel Prize for his work with the polymerase chain reaction [PCR] used in HIV detection said, "If there is evidence that HIV causes AIDS, there should be scientific documents that either singly or collectively demonstrate that fact, at least with a high probability. There is no such document."

And Dr. Heinz Ludwig Sanger, Emeritus Professor of Molecular Biology and Virology, Max Planck Institute of Biochemistry, Munich, said that it had become obvious that "Up to today there is actually no single scientifically really convincing evidence for the existence of HIV. Not even once such a retrovirus has been isolated and purified by the methods of classical virology."

The meticulous research of the Perth Group best summed things up:

> "What we are doing and have been doing from the very beginning is to question the accepted cause of AIDS and to put forward an alternative theory for the cause of AIDS which has a number of well-defined predictions, most of which have been satisfied."[15]

> "Since in our view at present no evidence exists that AIDS is caused by a retrovirus, we see no reason for AIDS patients to be treated with antiretroviral drugs. We did write a critical analysis on the use of AZT as an antiretroviral agent when we showed that, given its pharmacological properties, it is not possible for it to have an antiretroviral effect. We have also presented evidence that AZT and nevirapine do not prevent mother-to-child transmission. However, we never advised that antiretroviral drugs should never be prescribed, since up till now the possibility had not been excluded that they may have clinical benefits acting by means other than as antiretroviral agents. However, given the latest publication on HAART, this may not be the case."

The view of this publication is that what is called "HIV" is in reality viral forms of cell-wall-deficient (with either cell-wall defects or little or no cell wall at all) atypical tuberculosis complicating a picture of earlier exposure and acquisition of a tubercular infection, active or latent. Such virus-like cell-wall-deficient forms are the favored forms of TB and always have been. Such previous tubercular infection could have occurred at any time in the life of an individual, and most often does so in the formative years. But when existing tubercular infection, dormant or otherwise, is then coupled with exposure to an extremely virulent atypical tubercular forms (such as *M. avium*) commonly found in US AIDS, this deadly one-two punch of immunosuppression sets the stage for the so-called "opportunistic" infections that also jump on board in AIDS. Furthermore, if the antiretrovirals have any benefit toward the extension of the life of an AIDS patient, which some reports claim is on average 15 years, this has little to do with their action against "HIV" and a lot to do with the fact that such antiretrovirals, through mechanisms still being worked out, serve to suppress the two leading causes of infectious death in AIDS: *Mycobacterium tuberculosis* and *Mycobacterium avium*. It will also be shown that even the use of these antiretrovirals is apparently still not enough to prevent tubercular pathogens from being the leading cause of death, even in societies with free access to such HIV antiretrovirals.[16]

REFERENCES

1. CDC. Monitoring selected national HIV prevention and care objectives by using HIV surveillance data—United States and 6 US-dependent areas—2011. *HIV Surveillance Supplemental Report*. October 2013; 18(5).
2. Ho DD, Neumann AU, Perelson AS, Chen W, Leonard JM, Markowitz M. Rapid turnover of plasma virions and

CD4 lymphocytes in HIV-1 infection. *Nature.* 1995, 373: 123–126.
3. Kirk O et al. Infections with *Mycobacterium tuberculosis* and *Mycobacterium avium* among HIV-infected patients after the introduction of highly active antiretroviral therapy. *Am J of Respiratory and Critical Care Medicine.* 2000; 162: 865–872.
4. John JJ, Kaur A. Tuberculosis and HIV infection. *Lancet* 1993; 342(2): 676.
5. Welch K, Finkbeiner W. Autopsy findings in the acquired immune deficiency syndrome. *JAMA.* 1984; 252: 1152–1159.
6. Kiehn TE, Edwards FF. Infections caused by Mycobacterium avium complex in immunocompromised patients: diagnosis by blood culture and fecal examination, antimicrobial susceptibility tests, and morphological and seroagglutination characteristics. *J Clin Microbiol.* 1985; 21: 168–173.
7. Buchacz K, Baker RK, Palella FJ Jr, et al. AIDS-defining opportunistic illnesses in US patients, 1994–2007: a cohort study. *AIDS.* 2010; 24: 1549–59.
8. Bisburg E. Central nervous system tuberculosis with the acquired immunodeficiency syndrome and its related complex. *Ann Intern Med.* 1986; 105: 210–213.
9. Constantine NT, Callahan JD, Watts DM. Retroviral testing: essentials for quality control and laboratory diagnosis. Boca Raton, Florida: CRC Press; 1992:117–118.
10. Kashala O, Marlink R, Ilunga M, et al. Infection with human immunodeficiency virus type 1 (HIV-1) and human T cell lymphotropic viruses among leprosy patients and contacts: correlation between HIV-1 cross-reactivity and antibodies to lipoarabinomannan. *J Infect Dis.* 1994; 169: 296–304.

11. Barbaro G, HIV infection, highly active antiretroviral therapy and the cardiovascular system *Cardiovascular Res.* 2003; 60: 87–95.
12. Montagnier L. *Virus.* New York: WW Norton & Company, Inc.; 2000.
13. Zakowski P, Fligiel S. Disseminated Mycobacterium avium-intracellulare infection in homosexual men dying of acquired immunodeficiency. *JAMA.* 1982; 248: 2980–2982.
14. Lai KK, Stottmeier KD, Sherman IH, McCabe WR. Mycobacterial cervical lymphadenopathy: relation of etiologic agents to age. *JAMA.* 1984; 251:1286–1288.
15. Papadopulous-Eleapulos E, Turner VF. The Perth group challenges John Moore. *Rethinking AIDS* September 23, 2006. http://www.rethinkingaids.com/challenges/Moore-Perth.html.
16. Saraceni V et al. Tuberculosis as primary cause of death among AIDS cases in Rio de Janeiro, Brazil. *Int. J. Tuberc Lung Dis.* 2008; 12(7): 769–772.

1/EPIDEMIC

Manhattan, 1979:

By 1979, doctors in Manhattan began to notice a strange new disease killing what had been up to then healthy gay men. As reports mounted, the Centers for Disease Control (CDC) was forced to circulate similar notices of homosexual men in New York and Los Angeles with a weakened immune system dying from heretofore rare causes.[1]

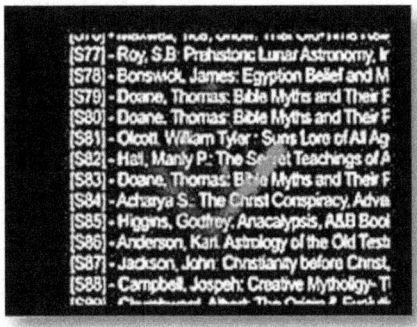

Figure 11. The First AIDS Cases Were Uncovered in Manhattan in 1979.

From its conception, AIDS was a nightmare of anguished victims, washed with wave after wave of terrible disease, whose physicians, like so many medical priests, helplessly watched them die. US coastal hospitals in San Francisco, New York, and Los Angeles soon turned into war zones.

The strange disease lurked among the gay habitual visitors of bathhouses. Men began dying of pneumonia and other respiratory illnesses, but only after drastically losing weight and developing horrific skin lesions on their faces, necks, backs, and chests. This disease became known in the gay community as "gay cancer." It was particularly volatile, and it progressed rapidly.

As more cases of the mysterious killer emerged, the name was changed from gay cancer to "gay-related immune deficiency" (GRID). This, at least, was an open recognition that whatever was causing the disease was compromising the body's immune system. It didn't explain, however, the rather esoteric choice of gay men, and soon to be discovered IV drug users as victims. Gay men realized the danger. Many made the intuitive leap early that perhaps certain activities, such as anal intercourse, might be transmitting the causative agent.

Rare diseases like *Pneumocystis carinii*, a tiny one-celled protozoa, filled gay lungs to the point of suffocation and requests for pentamidine aerosol to combat *Pneumocystis* trickled, and then poured, into the CDC. Another uncommon killer, Kaposi's sarcoma (KS) of the skin, became the most common form of this gay-related immune deficiency.

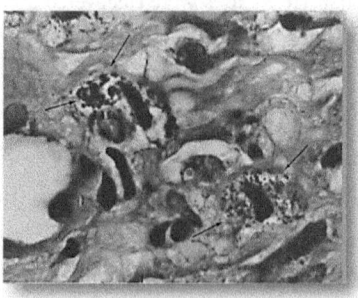

Figure 12. Kaposi's Sarcoma. Black arrows point to rounded tubercular microbes shaped as round cocci and granules in the tissue.

That AIDS could be sexually transmitted was incontrovertible, based on the gay sexual activities of Gaëtan Dugas alone. Dugas, a French Canadian air steward, was responsible for infecting at least 40 men either himself or through other men who had had contact with him. And of the 248 cases known before the detection of the virus, in excess of 40 of these AIDS victims had direct or indirect contact with Gaëtan Dugas. Dugas, who was on a collision course with history, only became sexually active in 1972. Born February 20, 1953, he would soon acquire the infamous name Patient Zero.

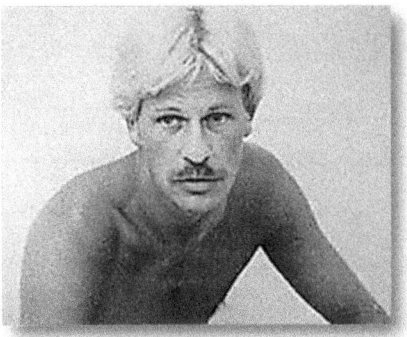

Figure 13. Gaëtan Dugas. At one point he was said to be patient zero of the North American AIDS pandemic.

On October 31, 1980—ominously enough, Halloween night— Gaëtan Dugas visited a gay bathhouse for the first time on a layover in New York City. It is speculated that Dugas caught the disease first there. Sometime later, after having casual sex in a darkened room, a male interviewee later reported that when he had turned on a light in the room where Dugas lay, he spotted the skin lesions (Kaposi's sarcoma) that were the classic earmarks of "gay cancer" on Dugas's chest. When he remarked about it, Dugas replied sardonically, "Its gay cancer. Maybe you'll get it." And so Gaëtan Dugas, the narcissistic and embittered flight attendant, was given the code name "Patient Zero", though he was indeed not the first to contract AIDS. But AIDS now had a face.

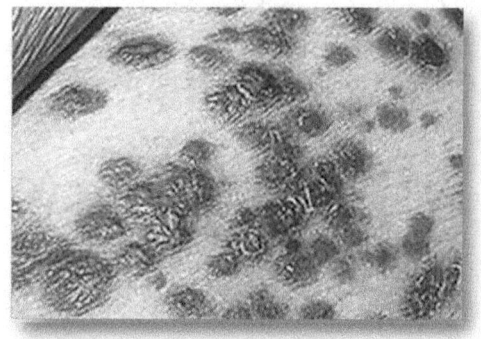

Figure 14. Kaposi's Sarcoma, Papular Type.

Nor was it only gays at risk. Drug addicts sharing needles, and hemophiliacs given pooled clotting factor VIII from blood so they would not bleed to death, soon became prey, also developing Kaposi's sarcoma and pneumocystis pneumonia. America's entire blood supply was in jeopardy, for by the early 1980s, gay and bisexual men accounted for one in four American blood donors.

AIDS throttled the immune system, in some cases shutting it down, and the primary site of attack always seemed traceable to the body's T-cells, white blood cell lymphocytes that held the body's invaders at bay.

By 1977, much evidence indicated that the basis of cellular immunity was tied in with T-cell lymphocytes—colorless, motile, cellular elements in the lymph. Chief in importance among these is the T-helper or CD4 lymphocyte, which fights infection. It soon became apparent that in AIDS, CD4 cells were either severely depleted, or they fell off the blood map altogether.

Panic-stricken virologists and other epidemiologists worked feverishly to isolate the source of this sexually transmitted disease whose first endemic wave washed up on American homosexual men's shores. Without delay, these same virologists, who for decades had failed miserably to find a retroviral cause for cancer, pounced on AIDS, dismissing any possibility other than a virus or a retrovirus, ignoring that it could just as easily be either one or a combination of older microbes presenting in a new way. Among them—Robert Gallo and Luc Montagnier.

Virologists initially told physicians to pass on the word that it was the cytomegalovirus that caused AIDS. Doctors dutifully obeyed, not fully realizing that all people, with time, are infected with cytomegalovirus.

Epidemiologist/retrovirologist Donald Francis, who would direct laboratory efforts for AIDS at the CDC and was also assistant director of the CDC's Division of Viral Diseases, had his own peculiar theory. Oddly enough, it was one also shared with epidemiologist James Curran, eventual director for AIDS research at the CDC. It went like this: Combine hepatitis with feline leukemia in cats—a retrovirus on which Francis wrote his doctorate—and you had Kaposi's sarcoma and the opportunistic infections seen in AIDS. Or maybe, just maybe, it was a retrovirus similar to the cat retrovirus—which in and of itself was solely responsible. Curran and Francis had worked together years ago developing the hepatitis B vaccine. They had all the connections in the scientific world that they needed.

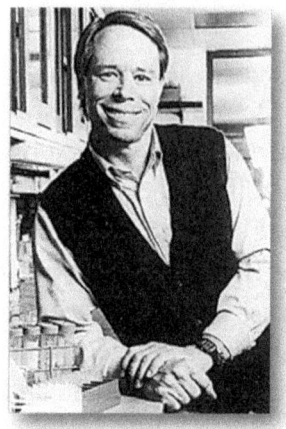

Figure 15. Donald P. Francis, MD, DSc.

Francis, one of the few at CDC who had actively wiped out smallpox worldwide, was considered an expert on both epidemics—and the cat leukemic virus. He would now combine his fields of 'expertise', quickly concluding that AIDS was cat leukemia in people. It was an impulsive long shot, and by most treated as such—at least initially.

REFERENCES
1. MMWR. *Morb Mortal Weekly Rep.* 1981; 30: 250–2.

2/CATS

In the Europe and the United States of the early eighties, a viral AIDS witch-hunt was on, and a few retrovirologists, strategically located at the CDC, National Institutes of Health (NIH), and the Harvard School of Public Health, joined ranks to force-feed a new option, a retrovirus.

William Jarrett, a veterinarian from the University of Glasgow, reported a "virus-like particle" associated with cat leukemia[1], but also found in many healthy cats. The particle would come to be called feline (cat) leukemic virus or FeLV. Or alternatively, it could be called the Jarrett virus leukemia,[1] allegedly a retrovirus that with time seemed to provoke malignant change, prevent cell development, and moreover cause immunosuppression in cats.[2,3] Most veterinarians did not speculate about the cause of human illness,—for obvious reasons. But this standard was soon breeched when Jarrett and his brother Oswald collaborated with Myron "Max" Essex and William Hardy to further study FeLV. Soon veterinarian-turned-retroviral researcher Myron "Max" Essex, doing further "cat house" studies at Harvard, saw what he felt was a parallel between feline leukemic virus and what was happening in human AIDS. He discussed his findings with Dr. Robert Gallo. Veterinarian Essex was one of the first to make the improbable assertion that since a "retrovirus," according to him, could cause immunosuppressive disease in cats, he also suspected that a retrovirus was the cause of AIDS. Retrovirologist Gallo was all ears.

Thus the possibility of an AIDS retrovirus, eventually called "HIV", was born, from a shaky leap in imagination that what Essex and Jarrett had found earlier in cats was now happening in humans.

In the background, Jane Teas, another researcher, who like Essex, was from the Harvard School of Public Health, deduced that AIDS was due to the African swine flu virus [ASFV].[4] Teas however, would be quickly drowned out by the retroviral cat fanciers.

The holes in the cat retroviral theory were enormous. Not only was it commonly found in normal healthy cats,[5] but the retrovirus was not present at all in one-third of cancerous cats.[6] Why one-third of malignant cats had no virus was unclear to everyone except the retroviral researchers who were certain that the cancer was still being caused by FeLV. As if this wasn't stretching the limits of credibility enough, Rogerson countered with the estimate that at least 50-60% of cats, or more at some point, became naturally infected by feline leukemic virus,[7] yet Dorn showed that only approximately 0.4% of all cats developed leukemia annually in their traditionally short lives.[8] In the United States today, an average of approximately 2-3%, on the average, of all cats are infected with FeLV.

Although these animal scientists spoke of AIDS caused by "an infectious agent, presumably a virus", their continued bombardment of the media about a feline leukemia/lymphoma virus that few medical doctors understood spoke with more certainty than presumption, and as Essex and his cat experiments faded, National Cancer Institute (NCI) retrovirologist Robert Gallo took up the banner in the form of his own leukemic/lymphomic human retroviruses, HTLV-1 and HTLV-2.

During it all, few realized that latent retroviruses were the most common nonpathogenic (non-disease-causing) viruses in either healthy animals or humans and were frequent harmless passenger viruses in not only AIDS, but cat, cow and human leukemia as well.[5]

Even before Koch discovered the causative organism of human tuberculosis in 1882, it was recognized in dogs and cats.[9] Up to 13% of cats[10] harbored the disease, often unsuspected. In most it spread to the lymph nodes, but it could also enter the cat's genital tract, in which case it assumed the capacity to become a sexually transmitted disease.[11] Often, a rapid course of cat death occurred, 10 — 20 days from the onset of symptoms.[10]

Recognized by Jordan[12] again in 1994, cat tubercular and mycobacterial infection had, like all mycobacteria, retroviral-like "cell-wall-deficient" or "L-forms", that could immunosuppress the animal to the point where other "opportunistic" diseases could arise in the cat[13]— and could also simulate cancer in a cat.[14]

It soon also became obvious that cats were also susceptible to *avium* tuberculosis, a leading cause of infection and death in American AIDS.[12,15,16]

By 1978, just prior to the recognition of the AIDS epidemic, Robert Gallo, isolating a human retrovirus from T-cell leukemia in the blood of a cancer patient, named it HTLV-1.

Problem was, it didn't cause the leukemia from which it was isolated [Sezary T-cell leukemia], only appeared in a small fraction of such cases, and was found in many, many healthy people.

HTLV-1 was now a retrovirus without a disease. But soon Gallo and colleagues, Max Essex among them, would suggest it as the probable cause of AIDS. Never mind that its prevalence in AIDS was no more than 25% and that just finding antibodies for it in AIDS blood was a hit-or-miss affair.

As it turned out, the retrovirus HTLV-1, despite the voluminous studies that validated it, did not cause AIDS. And now, the main fear of these cancer-turned-AIDS retrovirologists quickly became that their retrovirus would prove to be just another "opportunistic" infection, or worse yet, a "passenger" virus lurking behind the real cause of AIDS, something that the CDC was already preparing to report.[17] In fact at that point, Walter Dowdle, then chief of the CDC, concluded that based on existing facts, his center had put far too much time and emphasis into the retroviral hypothesis altogether.

That same year, however, French scientists, racing back from a New York AIDS symposium that spoke of a causal "human leukemic retrovirus" (HTLV) decided to enlist the help of retrovirologists at the famed Pasteur Institute. Pointing out the one true direction to go after a disease that destroyed the T-4 helper lymphocytes in the blood was to the lymph nodes themselves, they pursued retrovirologist Luc Montagnier, head of cancer virology, who had been looking for some time to blame cancer on a retrovirus. The fact that lymph nodes had been recorded to be a favored target of TB for centuries seemed to have completely escaped them. They had to validate a "retrovirus" in AIDS to compensate for their failed cancer efforts.

REFERENCES

1. Jarrett WFH, Crawford AM. Leukemia in the cat: a virus-like particle associated with leukemia [lymphosarcoma] *Nature.* 1964; 202: 566–568.
2. Jarrett O, Laird HM. Growth of feline leukemia virus in human cells. *Nature.* December 20, 1969; 224(225): 1208–9.
3. Jarrett O, Laird HM. Growth of feline leukemia virus in human, canine and porcine cells. *Bibl Haematol.* 1970; 36: 387–92.
4. Teas, J. Could AIDS agent be a new variant of African swine fever? *Lancet.* April 23, 1983; 1(8330): 923.
5. Duesberg PH Retroviruses as carcinogens and pathogens: expectations and reality. *Cancer Research.* March 1987; 47: 1199–1220.
6. Francis DP, Cotter SM. Comparison of virus positive and virus-negative cases of feline leukemia and lymphoma. *Cancer Research.* 1979; 39: 3899.
7. Rogerson P, Jarrett W. Epidemiological studies of feline leukemia virus infection. *Intl J. Cancer.* 1975; 15: 781–85.
8. Dorn CR, Taylor D. Cancer morbidity in dogs and cats from Alameda County. *J. Natl Cancer Instit.* 1968; 40: 307–18.
9. Blaine DP. Tuberculosis in the dog, cat and bird. *Vet Rec.* 1913; 25: 677.
10. Snider WR. Tuberculosis in canine and feline populations. *Am Rev of Resp Dis.* 1971; 104(6): 877–87.
11. Robin V, Brion A. Genital tuberculosis in a cat. *Rec Med Vet.* 1954; 130: 213.
12. Jordan HL. Disseminated *Mycobacterium avium complex* infection in three Siamese cats. *Am Vet Med Assoc.* January 1994; 204(1): 90–3.

13. Drolet R. Disseminated tuberculosis caused by *Mycobacterium avium* in a cat. *J. Am Vet Med Assoc.* November 15, 1986; 189(10): 1336–7.
14. Miller MA, Fales WH. Inflammatory pseudotumor in a cat with cutaneous mycobacteriosis. *Vet Pathol.* March 1999; Mar 36(2): 161–3.
15. Hix JW, Jones TC. Avian tubercle infection in the cat. *J Amer Vet Med Assoc.* 1961; 138: 641.
16. Malik R, Gabor L. Subcutaneous granuloma caused by *Mycobacterium avium complex* infection in a cat. *Aust Vet J.* 1998; Sep. 76(9): 604–7.
17. CDC update: Acquired immunodeficiency syndrome (AIDS)—United States. *Morb Mortal Weekly Rep.* 1983; 32:465–7.

3/CANCER STRUGGLES

America, Turn of the Century:

Indeed, the history of retroviruses mirrored cancer research.

In 1904, Ellermann and Bang, searching for an infectious bacterial cause for chicken leukemia,[1] succeeded in transferring it from one fowl to another by injecting cell-free tissue infiltrates. They sought a bacteria, but simply because it passed through a filter, the responsible agent was assumed to be a virus.

That same year, the first lentivirus, later claimed to be related to HIV, was isolated as a filterable equine infectious agent in horses by Valle and Carre at the Pasteur Institute.[2] Yet Peyton Rous, an authority on "invisible microbes", shrugged off Valle and Carre's filterable finding as no more than "small bacteria."[3]

Most authorities now realize that there are some viruses almost as large as bacteria and some bacteria as small as viruses, forms of which can easily pass through filters. This realization was quickly disputed by HIV enthusiasts Francis et al.[4] when they incorrectly said, "Since the infectious agent had obviously passed through a filter, it had to be a virus."

It did not.

Peyton Rous was credited with the discovery and isolation of the first retrovirus. By 1911, Rous wanted to know why if one chicken got cancer, others followed.⁵ Rous, who reproduced the tumor at will in Plymouth Rock fowls, favored a bacterial cause over a filterable virus. However, it was a question that he never definitely answered.

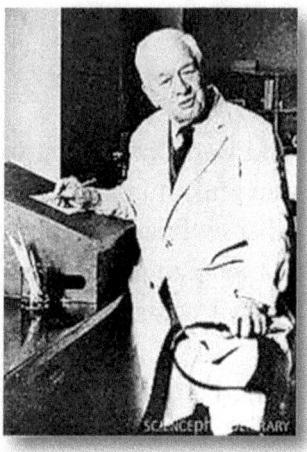

Figure 16. Dr. Francis Peyton Rous (1897–1970).

By 1933, Shope reported a viral tumor in cottontail rabbits, and Bittner reported on a milk-borne mouse breast cancer attributed to still another virus.⁶

In fact, by the 1950s, and with the advent of the electron microscope, particles later questionably ascribed to retroviruses were readily and routinely being detected. As a result, at a time when established medicine had about-faced and was now firmly set against an infectious cause for cancer, two controversial minority camps splintered from the mainstream, each diametrically at odds.

There were the virologists, who claimed that cancer was viral or retroviral, and another group whose careful, peer-reviewed research demonstrated that the retroviruses in the Rous, Bittner, and Shope tumors were actually filterable forms of mycobacteria.[7] Tuberculosis-like, these "viruses" could be stained with acid-fast dyes and readily passed through a filter, but they actually were a class of bacteria having many of the characteristics of mycobacteria such as tuberculosis.

This last-mentioned work, spearheaded by physician-researcher Virginia Livingston of Rutgers,[8] validated earlier work done by her proving that Rous's virus was a bacteria.[9,10] Soon others would join[11,12,13] Livingston's network, questioning the very existence of retroviruses, and the retrovirologists did not like it. A scientific life-and-death cancer struggle ensued.

By 1960, biologist-turned-retrovirologist Howard Temin sought to contrive an explanation for his observation as to why retroviruses, composed of RNA, Rous's among them, were inhibited by actinomycin D—an antibiotic and known bacterial DNA inhibitor. Based on this finding, Temin elaborately hypothesized the concept of reverse transcription with its "reverse transcriptase". But in truth, since antibiotics did not affect viruses, Temin's observation regarding the antibiotic actinomycin D's inhibition of the Rous retrovirus still made more sense if the Rous retrovirus was bacterial to begin with. It was later shown that Temin's reverse transcriptase was also utilized by other microbes, including *Mycobacterium tuberculosis*.

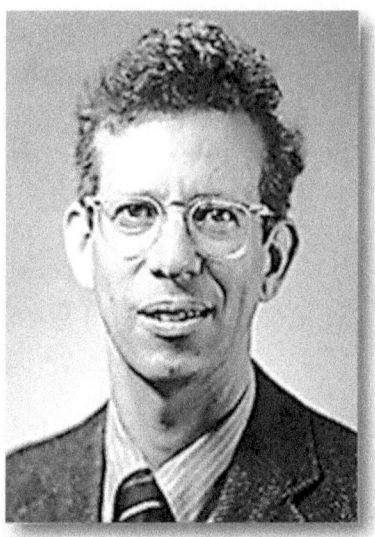

Figure 17. Howard M. Temin, PhD

Nevertheless, quickly capitalizing on the flawed logic of Temin, cancer viral investigators of the 1960s and 1970s reacted by conveniently misinterpreting his nonspecific enzyme discovery (reverse transcriptase), which in fact arose primarily as a function of normal cellular healing—and could be found in other pathogens—as a primary indicator for the newly scrutinized retroviruses. It was as a direct result of Temin's enzyme that 'oncoviruses', purported to cause cancer, suddenly became known as 'retroviruses'.

It was to Rutger's mycobacterial researcher Virginia Livingston's solid disadvantage that when Richard Nixon signed his National Cancer Act on December 23, 1971, he placed virologist Frank J. Rauscher Jr. as director of the newly established National Cancer Program (NCP).

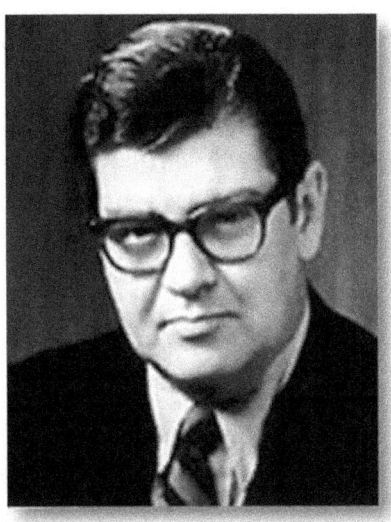

Figure 18. Frank J. Rauscher Jr.

With Rauscher at the controls, it was only a matter of time before cancer virologists, retrovirologists, and immunologists were pushed to the vanguard of America's War on Cancer. Once entrenched, they would remain at the helm even as, incredibly, their failed cancer attempts now turned toward finding the retroviral cause for AIDS.

Bacterial L-forms, the connecting link between viruses and bacteria, were first described by Emy Klieneberger at England's Lister Institute, for which she named them "L-forms." Such bacteria were 'cell-wall deficient' (CWD) because they either had a disruption in or a lack of a rigid bacterial cell wall. This lack of rigidity allowed them the plasticity to assume many forms (pleomorphic), some of them virus-like, but all of them different from their classical parent. Such forms were also poorly demonstrated by ordinary staining,[14] many of them, just like viruses, easily passing through the finest of filters. Of all the bacteria, it is tubercular L-forms (cell-wall-deficient forms) that predominate and are crucial to the survival of tuberculosis and the mycobacteria. It is mostly in its cell-wall-deficient forms that TB can escape destruction by the body's immune system. And at the same time, CWD forms of the tuberculosis-like mycobacteria react similarly in ELISA blood tests[15] to the 'HIV retrovirus', which they can simulate in every way.

Some years later, when HIV discoverer Luc Montagnier was interviewed for a French AIDS documentary, film-maker Djamel Tabi asked how he had isolated HIV. Incredibly, Montagnier's reply was that he did not isolate HIV, he just found something that looked like a retrovirus.[16]

Klieneberger, as well as Livingston, also saw parallels between the filterable forms of tuberculosis and 'mycoplasmic-like forms,' because without intact cell walls, the mycobacteria were often mistaken for the virus-like bacteria mycoplasma, which has no cell wall.[14] The differentiation between mycoplasma and cell-wall-deficient mycobacteria, reported Mattman, was difficult at best.[15]

REFERENCES

1. Ellermann V, Bang O. Experimentelle Leukamie bei Huhnern. *Zbt Bakt* 1908; 46: 595–609.
2. Vallee H, Carre H. Nature infectieuse de l'anemie du chevale. *CR Acad Sci*. Paris 1904; 139: 331–333.
3. Roux E. Sur les microbes dits inviibles. *Bull Inst Pasteur* 1903; 1: 7–12, 49–56.

4. Francis DP, Curran JW, Essex M. Epidemic acquired immune deficiency syndrome: epidemiologic evidence for a transmissible agent. *J Natl Cancer Inst.* 1983; 71: 1–4.
5. Rous PA. Sarcoma of the fowl transmissible by an agent separable from the tumor cells. *J Exp Med.* 1911; 13: 397–411.
6. Bittner JJ. Some possible effects of nursing on the mammary gland tumor incidence of mice. *Science.* 1936; 84: 162.
7. Livingston V. *Cancer: A New Breakthrough.* Los Angeles: Nash Publishing; 1972.
8. Livingston VA. Specific type of organism cultured from malignancy: bacteriology and proposed classification. *Ann NY Acad Sci.* 1970; 174: 636–654.
9. Duran-Reynals F. Neoplastic infection and cancer. *Am J Med.* 1950; 8(4): 440–511.
10. Glover T, Scott MA. Study of the Rous chicken sarcoma no. 1. *Canada Lancet and Practitioner* 1926; 66(2): 49–62.
11. Diller I. Donnelly experiments with mammalian tumor isolates. *Ann NY Acad Sci.* 1970; 174(2): 655–674.
12. Alexander-Jackson E. A specific type of microorganism isolated from animal and human cancer: bacteriology of the organism. *Growth.* 1954; 18: 37–51.
13. Seibert FB, Feldman RL. Morphological, biological, and immunological studies on isolates from tumors and leukemic bloods. *Ann NY Acad Sci.* 1970; 174(2): 690–728.
14. Klieneberger-Nobel E. Origin, development and significance of L-forms in bacterial cultures. *J Gen Microbiol.* 1949; 3: 434–442.
15. Mattman L. *Cell Wall Deficient Forms—Stealth Pathogens.* Boca Raton: CRC Press; 1993.
16. Null G. AIDS: a second opinion. *Townsend Letter for Doctors and Patients.* June 2000.

4/SHYH-CHING LO

Armed Forces Institute of Pathology, Washington, 1989:

Dr. Shyh-Ching Lo, MD, was a senior scientist at the prestigious, world-renowned Armed Forces Institute of Pathology in Washington. As he watched events unfold, and it became obvious that it was going to be dictum that HIV caused AIDS, he just had one problem. Whenever he examined someone who had died of AIDS, he could never find HIV, not even a trace of HIV-infected tissue damage. So Lo began his own search for an AIDS cause, which led him to a "virus-like infectious agent."[1] Knowing he was onto something, Shyh-Ching Lo followed his conscience, against the grain of most other scientists, and finally isolated not a virus but a mycoplasma. And in one study of 24 people with AIDS, he found antibody titers to it in practically everyone.[2] Shyh-Ching Lo would co-publish again, with Saillard.[3]

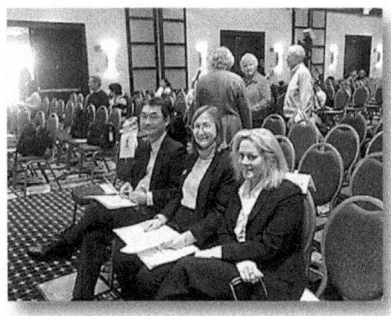

Figure 19. Shyh-Ching Lo, MD, About to Give a Presentation Regarding Recent Studies of the Epidemiology of MLV-Related Human Retroviruses.

That same year Livingston died, and a year later Luc Montagnier, the discoverer of HIV, almost got booed off a 1991 San Francisco podium by HIV activists at the Sixth International AIDS Conference—for endorsing Lo's mycoplasma as a necessary cofactor for the AIDS virus to become fatal.[4]

Montagnier and his colleague Lemaitre had done a hornet's nest of an experiment that put HIV activists on the edge of their chairs. In 1990, the two scientists published that cells cultured with 'HIV', which normally died, grew well in the presence of two antibiotics, minocycline and doxycycline.[5] Antibiotics do not affect retroviruses, so they were not working against HIV—it was a bacteria. Montagnier decided that that bacteria was probably Lo's mycoplasma. He had done so unaware of the fact that the two particular antibiotics he was using also had activity against Livingston's atypical tuberculosis.[6,7,8,9] In the meantime Nobel nominee Mattman made her claim that, even under the best of circumstances, it was difficult to differentiate certain mycoplasmas from cell-wall-deficient tuberculosis.

REFERENCES

1. Lo SC. Isolation and identification of a novel virus from patients with AIDS. *Am J Trop Med Hyg.* 1986; 35(4): 675–6.
2. Lo SC, Dawson MS. Identification of Mycoplasma incognito infection in patients with AIDS: an immunohistochemical, in situ hybridization and ultrastructural study. *Am J Trop Med Hyg.* 1989; 41(5): 601–616.
3. Saillard C, Carle P. Genetic and serologic relatedness between Mycoplasma fermentans strains and a mycoplasma recently

identified in tissues of AIDS and non-AIDS patients. *Res Virol.* 1990; 141(3): 385–395.
4. Ostrom N. Co-discoverer of AIDS virus says it may have microbial accomplice. *New York Native.* 1991; October 21.
5. Lemaitre M, Guetard D. Protective activity of tetracycline analogs against the cytopathic effect of the human immunodeficiency viruses in CEM cells. *Res Virol.* 1990; 141(1): 5–16.
6. Burns DN, Rohatgi PK. Disseminated Mycobacterium fortuitum successfully treated with combination therapy including ciprofloxin. *Am Rev Respir Dis.* 1990; 142(2): 468–470.
7. Gupta I, Kocher J. Mycobacterium haemophilum osteomyelitis in an AIDS patient. *N J Med* 1992; 89(3): 201–202.
8. Livingston V. *Cancer: A New Breakthrough.* Los Angeles: Nash Publishing; 1972.
9. Roussel G, Igual J. Clarithromycin with minocycline and clofazimne for Mycobacterium avium-intracellulare complex lung disease in patients without the acquired immune deficiency syndrome. GETIM. Groups d'Etude et de Traitement des Infections a Mycobceries. *Int J Tuberc Lung Dis.* 1998; 2(6): 462–470.
10. Tasaka S, Urano T. A case of *Mycobacterium fortuitum* pulmonary disease in a healthy young woman successfully treated with ciprofloxacin and doxycycline. *Kekkaku.* 1995; 70(1): 31–35.
11. Tsukamura, M. Chemotherapy of lung disease due to *Mycobacterium avium–Mycobacterium intracellulare* complex by a combination of sulfadimethoxine, minocycline, and Kitasamycin. *Kekkaku.* 1984; 59(1): 33–37.

Rutgers-Presbyterian Hospital Laboratory for the Study of Proliferative Diseases, Bureau of Biological Research, Rutgers University, New Jersey, 1950:

Livingston associate and prominent Cornell microbiologist Eleanor Alexander-Jackson,[1] a lifelong colleague, had a problem. As long as Alexander-Jackson held her reputation as one of the leading tuberculosis experts in the world, American medicine embraced her, but when she tried to attribute cancer to Livingston's tuberculosis-like germ, it would move to crush her.

Alexander-Jackson, whose advanced mycobacterial staining and culture techniques appeared in a 1944 issue of *Science*, carefully set a trap sure to ensnare virologists. The Rous virus, being a retrovirus, was supposed to be an RNA virus. So Alexander-Jackson knew that finding DNA in it would automatically mean that it was bacterial. It was understood that retroviral DNA should be present only in human or animal cells and nowhere else. But Alexander-Jackson's paper *Ultraviolet Spectrogramic Microscope Studies of Rous Sarcoma Virus Cultured in Cell Free Medium* demonstrated that there was DNA present in Rous, a characteristic of bacteria.[2] Why was it still being called a retrovirus?

When Livingston confronted Rous that his "retrovirus" could be dried, shelved, stored, and mixed months later in saline only to grow out on bacterial culture plates, he reminded her that he had never said it was a virus, carefully using the phrase "tumor agent."

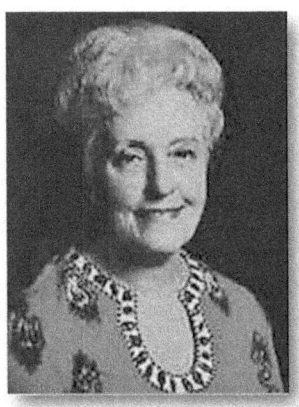

Figure 20. Virginia Livingston, MD

To be certain, the Livingston network concluded that oncogenic—supposedly cancer-causing—viruses were in fact L-forms of tuberculosis-like mycobacteria and related organisms. And Livingston was coming much too close to proving her point to suit American retrovirologists.

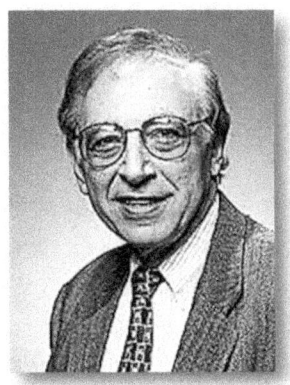

Figure 21. Dr. Robert Gallo

Threatened by Livingston and Alexander-Jackson's findings, HIV co-discoverer Robert Gallo huffed, "What is going on in this country? This is insanity! She can have her theories, and what can I say? I don't know of anything to support it. I can't see any basis, and I don't know what to say or what analogy to give you."[3]

No analogy required. Livingston's findings, with worldwide stature, were not about theories of retroviruses yet to be isolated. She had, in fact, come much closer than any of the retrovirologists in proving a direct causation between her organism and cancer by showing that her germ manufactured human growth hormone (HCG), long associated with malignancy.[4]

Before her death, Livingston would give one more clue towards unraveling what had become AIDS. There were "less known" and "little publicized" microorganisms that were transmitted sexually. Through bacteriological studies, she had confirmed that the very same L-forms of tubercular mycobacteria she found in Rous, by some called 'mycoplasma', could be found in the semen of man.[5]

REFERENCES

1. Alexander-Jackson EA. Specific type of microorganism isolated from animal and human cancer: bacteriology of the organism. *Growth.* 1954; 18: 37–51.
2. Alexander-Jackson EA. Ultraviolet spectrogramic microscope studies of Rous Sarcoma. *Ann NY Acad Sci.* 1970; 174(2): 765.

3. Parachini A. New "cure" for cancer stirs controversy. *Los Angeles Times.* April 6, 1984.
4. Livingston V, Wuerthele-Caspe, Livingston AF. Some cultural, immunological, and biochemical properties of progenitor cryptocides. Trans. *NY Acad Sci.* Ser II 1974; 36(6): 569–582.
5. Livingston V. *Cancer: A New Breakthrough.* Los Angeles: Nash Publishing; 1972.

5/IN THE SEMEN OF MAN

Although tuberculosis was, and still is, in scientific off-the-record fashion, rarely spoken of as a sexually transmitted disease, the not-uncommon potential for this has always existed. In the presence of prostatitis, it may be transmitted through the semen.[1]

As long as the mysterious killer behind AIDS remained comfortably within the gay community, not much was done to truly investigate it. As soon as AIDS found its way into the heterosexual population, though, suddenly America's interest in ferreting out the cause of AIDS became paramount.

Anyone who watched AIDS evolve—not only in gay America but heterosexually in Africa and Asia—could not help but be struck by its travel and spread along the epidemiologic highways of sex, drugs, migrants, prostitutes, bath houses, and venereal disease clinics. Yet the realization that sexual transmission of AIDS could occur between a man with risk factors and a woman came late.[2] Soon thereafter, female to male transmission, originally thought unlikely, was also found to occur.[3] By 1984, the pivotal importance female prostitutes played in the propagation of AIDS in equatorial Africa had become evident.[4]

But despite the magnifying forces of high-tech tests such as the polymerase chain reactors [PCRs], protein broths that make multiple copies of hard to find pathogens, its use in AIDS was never clear. Critics contested PCR in this situation, saying that it vastly exaggerates "HIV" by making numerous copies of fragments of nucleic acid, which might or might not even be HIV to begin with. And HIV itself could only be detected in a distinct minority of semen samples: one in twenty-five.[5]

On the other hand, ignored and unnoticed, the very real possibility of the genital transmission of *M. tuberculosis*, a disease affecting almost 2 billion people and intimately linked with and considered a reliable sign of AIDS,[6,7] as well as being frequently found in the genitourinary tract.[8]

REFERENCES

1. Lattimer JK, Colmore HP. Transmission of genital tuberculosis from husband to wife via the semen. *Am Rev Tuberc.* 1954; 69(4): 618–624.
2. Centers for Disease Control (CDC) Immunodeficiency among female sexual partners of males with acquired immune deficiency syndrome (AIDS)—New York. *Morb Mortal Weekly Rep.* 1983; 31: 700–1.
3. Piot P, Quinn TC. Acquired immunodeficiency syndrome in a heterosexual population in Zaire. *Lancet.* 1984; 2: 65–69.
4. Van de Perre P, Clumeck N. Female prostitutes: a risk group for infection with human T-cell lymphotropic virus type III. *Lancet.* 1985; 2: 524–526.
5. Van Voorhis BJ, Martinez A. Detection of human immunodeficiency virus type 1 in semen from seropositive men using culture and polymerase chain reaction deoxyribonucleic acid amplification techniques. *Fertile Steril.* 1991; 55: 588–594.
6. CDC. Tuberculosis—United States, 1985—and the possible impact of human T-lymphotropic virus type III/

lymphadenopathy associated virus infection. *Morb Mortal Weekly Rep.* 1986; 35: 74–6.
7. CDC. Diagnosis and management of mycobacterial infection and disease of persons with human immunodeficiency virus infection. *Ann Int Med.* 1987; 106: 254–6.
8. Wyngaarden JB, 19th ed. *Cecil Textbook of Medicine*; vol. 2. Philadelphia: WB Saunders, 1992:1740.

The Research Center for Genitourinary Tuberculosis, Kingsbridge Veterans Hospital, Bronx, New York, 1954:

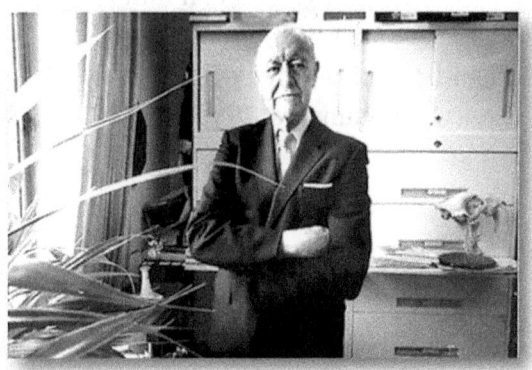

Figure 22. Dr. John K. Lattimer, MD. For 25 years, he was a professor and chairman of the urology department at the College of Physicians and Surgeons of Columbia University.

By 1954, a pattern had emerged at Dr. John Lattimer's Center for Genitourinary Tuberculosis. Men who developed tuberculosis epididymitis (inflammation of the testicles) were usually found to have an active focus of tubercular infection in their prostate, and cultures of their semen were frequently positive for tubercle bacilli.[1]

But while documenting sexual transmission, what puzzled John Lattimer most was why more husbands with prostatic TB were not infecting their wives. Two possibilities came to mind. First, the resistance of the thick, stratified vaginal epithelium to tubercular infection; second, the scorched earth policy of prostatic tuberculosis, whereby it sought to destroy glandular elements of the prostate,[1] severely decreasing semen volume. Many of his male patients, in fact, complained that orgasm produced only slight moisture at the tip of their penis, with over half of his experimental group having a semen volume of less than 0.5cc—too scanty to infect the vaginal or vulvar epithelium, if it reached them at all. As almost a testament to this finding—of 40 men with tuberculous genital infections, only one produced a child.[1]

Nevertheless, seeing sexual spread in a disease with staggering numbers right in front of him, Lattimer gave notice to the scientific world at large,[1] but few listened, and adequate descriptions of tuberculosis as a sexually transmitted disease never really reached medical texts. Curiously, despite this, tuberculosis is still often unofficially listed among or with the sexually transmitted diseases.

REFERENCES

1. Lattimer JK, Colmore HP. Transmission of genital tuberculosis from husband to wife via the semen. *Am Rev Tuberc.* 1954; 69(4): 618–624.

Niagara Peninsula Sanatorium, St. Catharine's, Ontario, Canada, December 1954:

Dr. Edgar T. Peer was more than a bit skeptical as he reviewed Lattimer's study regarding the seminal transmission of tuberculosis.

He himself had recovered tubercle bacilli from a patient's semen in 1952 but dismissed it as lab error. He would later write that like most dismissals of the tubercle bacilli on similar grounds, it would come back to haunt him.

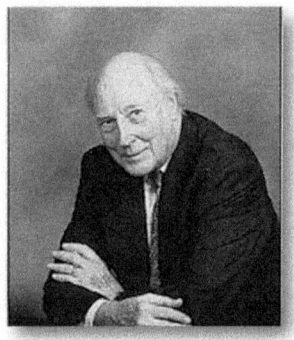

Figure 23. Edgar T. Peer, MD

By 1954, Peer's cases of sexually transmitted tuberculosis were mounting and, struck by similarities beyond coincidence, he saw an "extremely probable source" of tuberculosis coming from the male genital tract.

Peer published, warning that if physicians did not wake up to the possibility of sexually transmitted genital tuberculosis, its diagnosis would continue to be unsuspected and underestimated,[1] which one day could lead to potentially catastrophic consequences.

Nor were Peer and Lattimer alone. Netter mentioned that the spread of the tubercle bacilli through the female genital tract by coitus with a tuberculous male could not be denied.[2] In fact, wherever culture of the seminal fluid showed *Mycobacterium tuberculosis*, there was a possibility of transmission of genital tuberculosis from male to female via the semen through sexual intercourse.[3] While Lattimer[4] and Peer[1] showed that the development of tuberculous ulcers in the vagina or vulva resulting in swollen lymph nodes in the groin were due to semen-positive males harboring *M. tuberculosis*, Hellerstrom clocked the actual incubation period—from the date of coitus during which the wife was exposed to the development of a vaginal or vulvar ulcer and enlargement of inguinal lymph nodes—to approximately three to four weeks.[5]

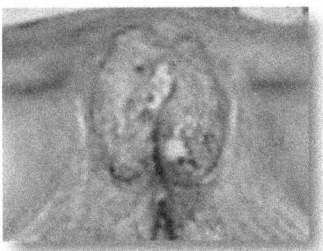

Figure 24. Tuberculosis of the Vulva.

Heins then offered a better idea of the potential potency of sexually transmitted mycobacteria such as tuberculosis, demonstrating that even the tame *Mycobacteria smegmatis*—found in the smegma of the genital secretions of every man and woman alive—when introduced into the vaginas of female mice resulted in the immediate death of over half of an experimental group of fourteen.[6]

Lattimer's cases were compiled from European and American literature. The ulcer and enlarged nodes in the female, often misdiagnosed, closely resembled lymphogranuloma inguinale, syphilis, or chancroid—all diseases that could coexist with tubercular sexually transmitted disease.[4]

And just as men could transmit mycobacterial tubercular disease to women, so too could women infect men.[7] By 1870, Soloweitschnick had documented the first observation of a tuberculous ulceration of the penis.[8]

Lewis cited 110 documented cases of tuberculosis of the penis written up before 1946. Twenty-nine additional cases were subsequently reported by Lal.[9] In his series of primary cases, Lewis pointed to 14 of venereal origin—12 penile ulcerations being definitely the result of coitus and two as a result of oral sex.[7]

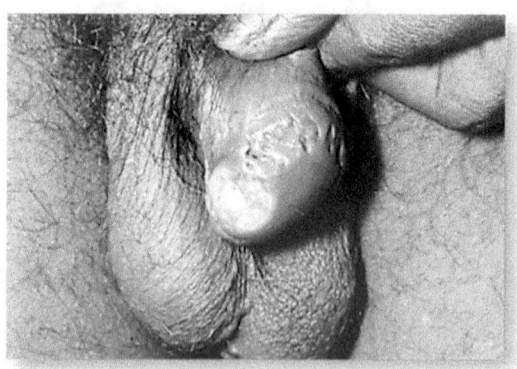

Figure 25. Penile ulcer from tuberculosis

Penile ulcers, newly attributed to primary HIV,[10] were already well documented in TB literature.[7,11,12,13] And the "giant cells" claimed to originate from HIV[14,15] were decades ago seen at the base of tubercular ulcers.[7] Long a hallmark of tuberculosis, multinucleated giant cells form in the tissues and engulf the tubercle bacilli in an attempt to kill them.[16]

Lewis mentions that of all the ways in which the penis could be infected with tubercle bacilli, direct contact was by far the most common. Although he documented transmission mostly through vaginal sex and occasionally oral sex, rectal transmission was not explored.[7]

To explain cases claimed not to arise from direct vaginal inoculation, woman to man, Lewis borrowed from Verneuil's hypothesis, somehow overlooked by later writers. In 1883, Verneuil, in *Hypothesis on the Origin of Genital Tuberculosis in the Two Sexes,* proposed a mechanism whereby men with infected urine or semen first inoculated the vaginal vault of their partners, and then, through subsequent sex, became themselves re-inoculated at the corona or frenulum of their own penises.[17] Years passed, but warnings persisted.

By 1972, five years before gays started dying in the United States, Rolland wrote[18] *Genital Tuberculosis, a Forgotten Disease?* And ironically, in 1979, on the eve of AIDS recognition, Gondzik and Jasiewicz showed that even in the laboratory, genitally infected tubercular male guinea pigs could infect healthy females through their semen by an HIV-compatible ratio of one in six, or 17%, prompting him to also warn his patients that not only was tuberculosis a sexually transmitted disease, but also the necessity of the application of suitable contraceptives such as condoms to avoid it.[19]

Gondzik's solution and pre-AIDS date of publication are chilling; his findings too significant to ignore. Even in syphilis at its most infectious stage, successful transmission in humans was possible only in 30% of contacts.[20]

Two years later, investigators in South Africa, itself perched on the precipice of its own devastating sexually transmitted AIDS epidemic, issued a report of 91 cases of tuberculosis of the penis.[21,22] This was followed by documentation in which 'HIV' in young African females came only after first contracting genital TB.[23]

Moreover, the fact that *Mycobacterium avium-intracellulare*, also known as fowl or swine tuberculosis and considered an "atypical" tuberculosis—could also act like a sexually transmitted disease, set up an explosive scenario.[24,25,26]

Avium had, in the short space of 30 years, gone from relative obscurity to the leading infectious disease in US AIDS. And despite the fact that DePaepe's group used only the conventional Ziehl-Neelsen tubercular stain without culture of either testicular tissue or semen, they still found *M. avium* in these specimens in 32% of AIDS patients with systemic *M. avium*—the same *M. avium* that would eventually kill most US AIDS patients who did not die from another AIDS-related disease.[27]

REFERENCES

1. Peer ET. Genitourinary transmission of tuberculosis. *Am Rev Tuberc.* 1957; 75: 153.
2. Netter FH. *Reproductive system. The Ciba Collection of Medical Illustrations.* New Jersey: West Caldwell, 1987; 2: 188.
3. Chakravarty SC, Sircar DK. Genital tuberculosis in males. Seminal fluid culture and vaso-seminal vesiculography studies. *J Indian Med Assoc.* 1968; 51(6): 283–286.
4. Lattimer JK, Colmore HP. Transmission of genital tuberculosis from husband to wife via the semen. *Am Rev Tuberc.* 1954; 69(4): 618–624.
5. Hellerstrom S. *Acta Dermato-Venereol.* 1937; 18(4): 465.
6. Heins Jr. HC, Dennis EJ. The possible role of smegma in carcinoma of the cervix. *Am J Obstet Gynecol.* 1958; 76: 726–735.
7. Lewis EL. Tuberculosis of the penis. Report of 5 new cases and complete review of the literature. *J Urol.* 1946; 56: 737.
8. Brunati J. Tuberculosis of the penis; surgical form-case. *Rev Chir,* Paris. 1937; 75: 213–233.
9. Lal DN, Sekhon GS. Tuberculosis of the penis. *J Indian Med Assoc.* 1971; 56: 316–318.
10. Hirschel B. In: Polsky, Clumeck, eds. *HIV and AIDS.* London: Mosby-Wolfe; 1999.
11. Jaisankar TJ, Bhagath RG. Penile Lupus vulgaris. *Int J Dermatol.* 1994; 33(4): 272–274.
12. Jeyakumar W, Ganesh R. Papulonecrotic tuberculids of the glans penis: case report. *Genitourin Med.* 1988; 64: 130–132.
13. Wood B. An unusual cause of penile ulceration. *South African Med J.* 1991; 79(1): 284.

14. Lifson JD, Reyes GR. AIDS retrovirus induced cytopathology: giant cell formation and involvement of CD4 antigen. *Science.* 1986; 232(4754): 1123–1127.
15. Popovic M. Detection, isolation and continuous production of cytopathic retroviruses (HTLV-III) from patients with AIDS and pre-AIDS. *Science.* 1984; 224(4648): 497–500.
16. Livingston V. *Cancer: A New Breakthrough.* Los Angeles: Nash Publishing; 1972.
17. Verneuil A. Hypothesis on the origin of genital tuberculosis in the two sexes. *Gaz Hebt d Med.* 1883; 25: 225.
18. Rolland R, Schellekens L. Genital tuberculosis, a forgotten disease. *Ned Tijdschr Geneeskd.* 1972; 116(52): 2377–2378.
19. Gondzik M, Jasiewicz J. Experimental study on the possibility of tuberculosis transmission by coitus. *Z Urol Nphrol.* 1979; 72(12): 911–914.
20. Smith LH, Wyngaarden JB. *Cecil Textbook of Medicine.* Philadelphia: WB Saunders; 1988.
21. Morrison JGL, Fourie ED. The papulonecrotic tuberculide: from Arthus reaction to Lupus vulgaris. *Br J Dermatol.* 1974; 91: 263–270.
22. Wilson-Jones E, Winkelmann RK. Papulonecrotic tuberculosis; a neglected disease in Western countries. *J Am Acad Dermatol.* 1986; 14: 815–826.
23. Giannacopoulos KC, Hatzidaki EG. Genital tuberculosis in an HIV infected woman. *Eur J Obstet Gynecol Reprod Biol.* 1998; 80(2): 227–229.
24. Damsker B, Bottone EJ. Mycobacterium avium–Mycobacterium intracellulare from the intestinal tracts of patients with the acquired immunodeficiency syndrome: concepts regarding acquisition and pathogenesis. *J Infect Dis.* 1985; 151(1): 179–181.

25. De Caprariis PJ, Giron JA. Mycobacterium avium-intracellulare infection and possible venereal transmission. *Ann Intern Med.* 1984; 101(5): 721.
26. De Paepe ME, Guerrieri C, Waxman M. Opportunistic infections of the testes in the acquired immunodeficiency syndrome. *Mt Sinai J Med.* 1990; 57(1): 25–29.
27. Nightingale SD, Byrd LT. Mycobacterium avium-intracellulare complex bacteremia in human immunodeficiency virus positive patients. *J Infect Dis.* 1992; 165: 1082–1085.

Queens Hospital Center, Long Island Jewish-Hillside Medical Center, Jamaica, New York, 1984:

Dr. Pascal De Caprariis saw before him a dying 30-year-old Haitian man with AIDS. A biopsy of the lymph node in the patient's groin showed *Mycobacterium avium-intracellulare* (fowl tuberculosis) seemingly gone systemic—spreading to the liver. Despite using different combinations totaling seven different antitubercular drugs, the patient died. If ever there was a harbinger of things to come, this was it.

Just before the patient's death, an ulcerative lesion of the corona of the penis formed. Tests for herpes were negative. Upon culture, and only upon culture, the *Mycobacterium avium*—or fowl tuberculosis so prevalent in US AIDS—was isolated from the penile crater, and De Caprariis started speculating that with this and his patient's right groin lymphatic swelling, sexual transmission of Avium (fowl tuberculosis) seemed neither farfetched nor improbable.[1]

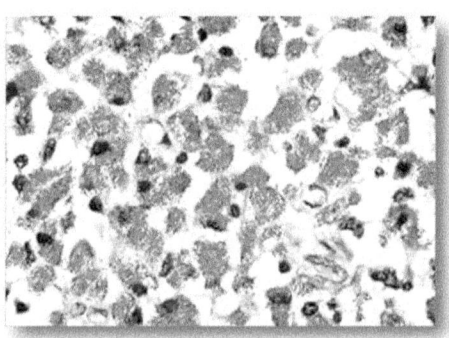

Figure 26. Mycobacterium avium in Lymph Node Tissue of an AIDS Victim.

REFERENCES

1. De Caprariis PJ, Giron JA. Mycobacterium avium-intracellulare infection and possible venereal transmission. *Ann Intern Med.* 1984; 101(5): 721.

Department of Microbiology, Mount Sinai Hospital, New York, 1985:

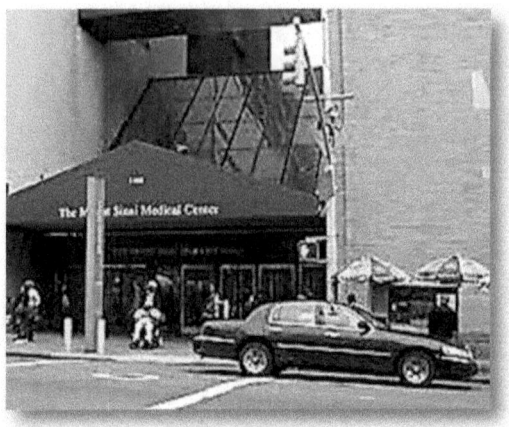

Figure 27. Mount Sinai Hospital in New York, NY

AIDS is what defined the decade of the 1980s, a decade that lived in fear beneath the partial shadow of a certain and tortuous death from a highly communicable pathogen.

But no one came closer to unlocking its true cause and mystery than American microbiologist Beca Damsker, MD. Damsker found overwhelming fowl tuberculosis infections of the colon and rectal tissues in US gay AIDS time and time again—and knew that an anorectal portal of transmission had to be considered important in its transmission. Damsker was also picking up fowl tuberculosis in the buffy coat of the blood of recently acquired AIDS victims—that fraction of an anticoagulated blood sample that contains most of the white blood cells and platelets following centrifugation.

Gay men instinctively realized the implications of Damsker's colon and rectal studies. Many had already made the intuitive leap that perhaps certain activities, such as anal intercourse, might be transmitting the causative agent. It was just that no one knew the specific agent being transmitted. Beca Damsker had just found that agent in fowl tuberculosis (*Mycobacterium avium*, or simply *M. avium*), but she had no way of knowing how universal the process she was examining really was in AIDS. But the regularity with which Damsker found *avium*, also known as swine tuberculosis, in gay stool and lower intestinal biopsy specimens, stunned even her.[1] Indeed, what Beca Damsker was seeing before her was a microcosm of the killer AIDS epidemic going on just outside her Mount Sinai research facility. Damsker's study was published in the *Journal of Infectious Diseases* in 1985.

Avium, or fowl tuberculosis, is a ubiquitous germ, found in animal reservoirs such as birds and pigs, among others.[2] As to how AIDS originated in man, Damsker was not unaware of the possibility that a small subset of homosexuals had a proclivity for bestiality—sexual activities with animals—a potential vector for virulent mycobacterial introduction with subsequent transmission to man, which when combined with the fragility of the paper-thin rectal mucosa to local trauma or intercourse and antigenic challenge,[3] could have led to calamitous unchecked multiplication of *M. avium* in gay AIDS, possibly of animal origin, in the intestinal mucosa and nearby lymph nodes. This then would have set the stage for AIDS to spread into the blood, with consequent targeting of other systems.[1] Beca Damsker already had all the evidence she needed.

Tuberculosis in swine is almost always caused by *M. avium*,[4] and such avian tuberculosis leads to some of the highest financial losses in the swine and poultry farm industry.[5]

Although the commonly found fowl tuberculosis was thought of as an "opportunistic" infection that occurred only late in the immunosuppression of AIDS, Damsker encouraged a closer look regarding the temporal relationship between fowl tuberculosis infection and the inception of American AIDS. In foreseeing this, Beca Damsker's assessment of what doctors were picking up late in the disease was to her nothing other than a stepwise advance and increment of its causal germ. And her reasoning seemed squarely on target. From a rectal portal of entry, the germ merely progressed in ferocity and immunosuppression as the disease advanced and lowered CD4 counts.[1] Indeed, Beca Damsker, in speculating about this, presented the single most plausible cause for American AIDS written to that point—and since.

REFERENCES

1. Damsker B, Bottone EJ. Mycobacterium avium–Mycobacterium intracellulare from the intestinal tracts of patients with the acquired immunodeficiency syndrome: concepts regarding acquisition and pathogenesis. *J Infect Dis.* 1985; 151(1): 179–181.
2. Chapman JS. *The Atypical Mycobacteria and Human Mycobacteriosis.* New York: Plenum Press; 1977.
3. Mavligit GM, Talpaz M. Chronic immune stimulation by sperm alloantigens. Support for the hypothesis that sperma-

tozoa induce immune dysregulation in homosexual males. *JAMA.* 1984; 251(2): 237–245.
4. Karlson AG. The incidence of tuberculosis in animals in the USA. *Bull Int Union Against Tuberc.* 1968; 40: 61–63.
5. Berthelsen JD. Economics of the avian TB problem in swine. *J Am Vet Med Assoc.* 1974; 164: 307–308.

6/THE TRAGIC COST OF PREMATURE CONSENSUS

Pasteur Institute, Paris, January, 1983:

The Pasteur Institute squeezed Luc Montagnier, the head of cancer virology, into the pressure cooker of finding an AIDS retrovirus when its production of a hepatitis B vaccine, accounting for a significant part of its income—in part processed from pooled American homosexual blood—came under fire.

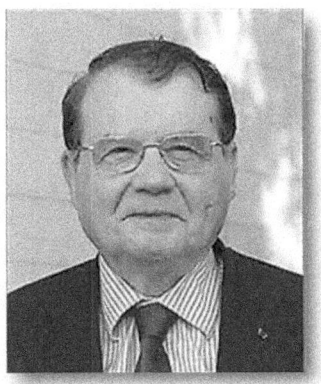

Figure 28. Dr. Luc Montagnier

Montagnier, on his part, was exclusively looking for a retrovirus related to Gallo's failed HTLV-1. He instead stumbled upon the retrovirus "LAV" which, in true wastebasket category fashion, stood for "lymphadenopathy-associated virus." How did he know it existed? Because his assistant Françoise

Barré-Sinoussi said that she found it…or at least she found something that looked like it.

LAV was so named because the French homosexual fashion designer from whom it was first isolated had enlarged, inflamed neck nodes (lymphadenopathy), a common early AIDS feature. Thirty-three and promiscuous, he had also visited New York City in 1979, and had a 50-gay-partners-a-year history.

Betting the obvious—that the agent responsible for AIDS could be more readily detected in these swollen lymph nodes—Barré, in January 1983, packed a small piece of the man's just-biopsied lymph node in ice at Paris's Pitie-Salpetriere Hospital and delivered it to Montagnier at Pasteur. This patient did not yet have full-blown AIDS, but his history and symptoms were strongly suggestive.[1] He would die five years later of the disease.

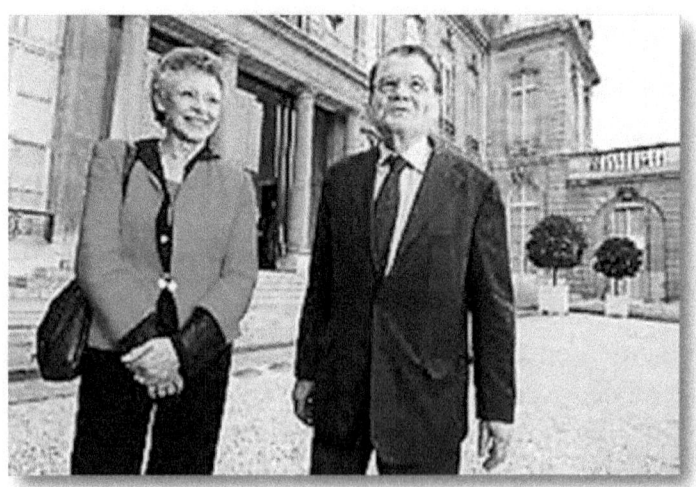

Figure 29. Montagnier and Barré-Sinoussi

At Pasteur, Montagnier put the tissue into cell cultures of T-lymphocytes. Immediately, questions arose as to the procedure. Looking only for a retrovirus, the team cultured whole-tissue lymph node lysates. The "virus" was never isolated in its pure form. It would be the beginning of a long, long line of research work based on indirect evidence.

Later, looking at Montagnier's tissue cultures microscopically revealed many granules, some of which were felt to look like retroviruses. But they were inside cells and tissues—not whole viral particles—and had different shapes and sizes. No two were alike. They seemed to show all forms of 'viral maturation', but were they viral?

As early as 1928, Eleanor Alexander-Jackson began discovering unusual—and to that point, unrecognized—forms of the TB bacillus. Jackson marveled at the many forms of tuberculosis, including the tiny granules that the German Hans Much saw in 1908, which soon became known as Much's granules.[4] In 1910, Fontes proved that Much's granules, as a subclassification of Kleinberger's L-forms, were filterable and therefore also often mistaken for viruses. In fact, in certain circles the variable acid-fast granules were called "the TB virus."[2]

But even prior to Livingston (1970), Mellon and Fisher had cautioned[3] that filterable forms of *M. avium* and human tuberculosis itself could easily be mistaken for the virus Montagnier and Barré thought they had and might explain what Mellon described as "the common finding by French workers of tubercular acid-fast bacilli in the glands of guinea pigs into which viral-like (cell-free) filtrates of tuberculosis material had been injected."[3]

REFERENCES
1. Barré-Sinoussi F, Chermann JC. Isolation of a T-lymphotropic retrovirus from a patient at risk for acquired immune deficiency syndrome (AIDS). *Science.* 1983; 220: 868–871.
2. Fontes A. Bemerkungen uber die Tuberkulose Infektion und ihr virus. *Mem Inst Oswaldo Cruz.* 1910; 2: 141–146.
3. Mellon RR, Fisher LW New studies on the filterability of pure cultures of the tubercle group of microorganisms. *J Infect Dis.* 1932; 51:117-128.4. Much H. Die Variation des tuberkelbacillus in form and wirkung. *Beitr Klim Tuberk.* 1931; 77: 60–71.

7/THE RACE

Pasteur Institute, Paris, 1983:

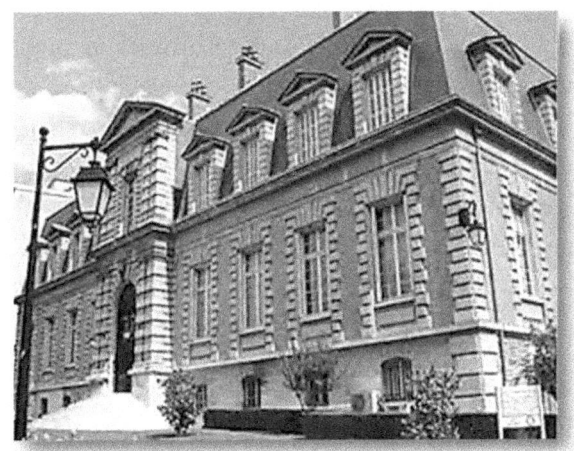

Figure 30. Institut Pasteur, Paris

Gallo's leukemic retrovirus (HTLV), which Barré and Montagnier thought they had isolated, should have led to the wild proliferation of lymphocytes. But all that Françoise Barré-Sinoussi found in subsequent trips to the lab was how well it was slaughtering them. This deeply disturbed her, as retroviruses typically didn't kill cells. How could she explain this?

By January 25, 1983, Barré-Sinoussi's reverse transcriptase radioactivity counter was clicking away with increased activity, which to her, as a retrovirologist, meant that her lymph node 'retrovirus', LAV, must be multiplying.

But reverse transcriptase is nonspecific and also found elevated in events leading to the death of CD4 lymphocytes by tuberculosis,[1] as well as in *M. avium* infection of neck lymph nodes,[2] probably the very event Françoise Barré-Sinoussi was watching. Again, why had she not considered these as possible AIDS causes?

In actuality, having previously been retroviral cancer researchers, Barré-Sinoussi and Montagnier were solely attuned, intellectually and technologically, to detecting "retroviruses". Barré had been trained in mouse retroviral techniques requiring the measurement of reverse transcriptase at Robert Bassin's National Cancer Institute (NCI) lab. Her procedures were not designed to explore for some unknown pathogen. In effect, Françoise Barré-Sinoussi and Luc Montagnier found a retrovirus because that was all that they were looking for.

Within weeks, Montagnier called a staff meeting. The new "retrovirus" wasn't Gallo's discredited HTLV-1, so everyone could breathe a sigh of relief. He also wasn't asserting that his retrovirus HAV actually caused AIDS, but it was possible. In the future, he would send samples of the tissue culture to Gallo, who headed AIDS research at NCI, to stimulate further research.

Approximately one year later, after receiving French samples from Montagnier, retrovirologist Gallo isolated and announced that he felt that his newly isolated HTLV-3 retrovirus must cause AIDS—a retrovirus that proved to be a carbon copy of Montagnier's LAV retrovirus, which Gallo said was a productive lentivirus infection with all forms of viral maturation.

A colleague had suggested on a hunch that Montagnier characterize his virus as a lentivirus ("lenti" means slow). Lentiviruses were large viruses which, after entering cells, did not leap into activity at once, but later shot into action. But so-called "slow viruses" had been implicated, but never proved, in diseases such as Creutzfeldt-Jakob, and Alzheimer's as well. Prominent American retrovirologist Peter Duesberg, who did much of the pioneer work on retroviral ultrastructure, knew that as direct pathogens, the retroviruses were not 'slow' viruses. They were not even lentiviruses like visna, with which HIV was often compared. Visna never acted like that. Rather, if visna reached high enough blood concentration, Duesberg related, it was rapidly pathogenic.[3] The human immunodeficiency virus (Gallo's HTLV-3 or Montagnier's HAV) however, was not to be found in such high amounts in the blood. Perplexed, Duesberg concluded that there was no such thing as a slow virus, "only slow virologists."[4] On the basis of his experience with retroviruses, Duesberg has challenged the virus-AIDS hypothesis in the pages of such journals as *Cancer Research, Lancet, Proceedings of the National Academy of Sciences,* and the *New England Journal of Medicine.*

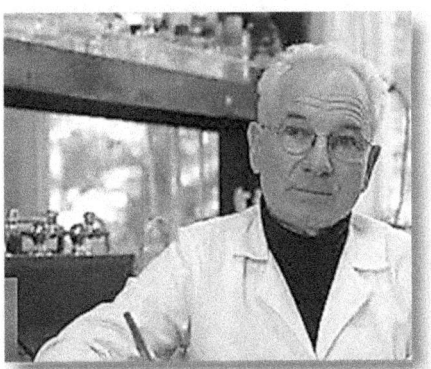

Figure 31. Peter H. Duesberg, PhD

The discovery of LAV (HIV) allowed virologists to worm their way into taking the high ground in American medicine. No longer would practicing physicians like Livingston, who had seen disease face-to-face, assume leadership on policy issues. The new medical shamans would be laboratory gene splicers, molecular biologists, virologists, and immunologists, who told doctors what to think about conditions they never had clinically treated. A dangerous precedent was being set.

REFERENCES

1. Watson E, Hill LL. Apoptosis in *Mycobacterium tuberculosis* infection in mice exhibiting varied immunopathology. *J Pathol.* 2000; 190(2): 211–2203.
2. April MM, Garelick JM. Reverse transcriptase in situ polymerase chain reaction in atypical mycobacterial adenitis. *Arch Otolaryngol Head Neck Surg.* 1996; 122(11): 1214–1218.
3. Lairmore MD, Rosadio RH. Ovine lentivirus lymphoid interstitial pneumonia. Rapid induction in neonatal lambs. *Am J Pathol.* 1986; 125: 173–181.
4. Health Education AIDS Liaison (HEAL), HIV 101: *10 Scientific Reasons Why HIV Cannot Cause Aids.* Toronto, 2001.

Cambridge University Clinical School, Cambridge, England, September, 1983:

Former viral cancer researcher Abraham Karpas worked out of the Department of Hematological Medicine at Cambridge. By September 1983, he had identified a "transmissible agent" through electron micrographs of the blood of a gay AIDS patient.[1]

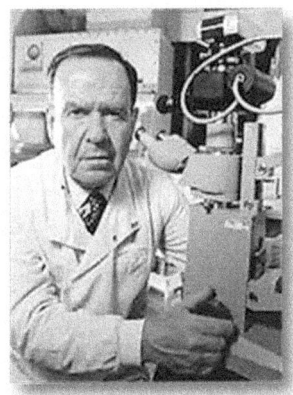

Figure 32. Dr. Abraham Karpas

Karpas was having a problem with Gallo's HTLV1 and was unable to confirm previous reports of this purported AIDS retrovirus in Africans. Many blood tests finding HTLV1 positive by previous investigators were found negative when retested in Karpas's lab.[2] Why was this happening?

Karpas, probably the second man in the world to see the AIDS agent, fired off a quick report on his transmissible agent, complete with a microphotograph, but he was having difficulty getting the paper published. He had the honesty to admit that he wasn't certain that the 55 nm particles with their 10 nm electrodense cores were viruses at all and began his paper with the phrase "Assuming it is a virus," though whatever it was, he later found it identical to Montagnier's "HIV."

Experts in the field sided with Karpas's restraint. Not only were retroviral particles "no proof that a virus was involved," but such particles were ubiquitous—a statement supported by O'Hara's Harvard study, which found "viral particles, morphologically indistinguishable" in 90% of the enlarged lymph nodes in both AIDS and non-AIDS patients.[3] O'Hara's study stood out as the one study to date that used suitable controls, finding 'viral particles' indistinguishable from HIV in a variety of swollen lymph nodes *without* HIV.

Similarly, African studies of the lymph nodes of patients with HIV also showed them to be indistinguishable from those with just tuberculosis and no AIDS.[4,5] O'Hara concluded, "The presence of such particles does not, by themselves, indicate infection with HIV." Yet it was the photomicrographs of these same particles that first informed the world that there was an HIV.

In *Reproduction of RNA Tumor Viruses*, Badar warned that *in vitro* cultures, even virus free, "can be induced to produce particles which resemble RNA tumor viruses in every physical and chemical respect,"[6] an event many saw as analogous to the rigors and harsh processes Montagnier and Gallo put their AIDS tissues through.

Oddly, it would not be until 1997 that two independent groups would examine these HIV particles in accordance with accepted international procedure.[7,8] Both teams saw an excess of fluid-filled, many-formed (pleomorphic) "contaminating" vesicles, ranging in size from 50 nm to 500 nm, as opposed to a minor population of particles of about 100 nm.

The latter were assumed to be viral, but proved, according to critics, to be too large, of the wrong shape, and containing too much material to be retroviruses. In fact, both the particles and vesicles of Bess and Gluschankof share common antigenic determinants with and could easily have been the variably acid-fast tubercular mycobacterial L-forms microphotographed by Seibert,[9] Alexander-Jackson,[10] Livingston,[11] and Cantwell.[12] Livingston showed a protoplast of tuberculosis with L-form inclusions budding out vesicles from its surface, not unlike the vesicles in the 1997 AIDS verification studies, while Seibert and Cantwell showed particles similar to those attributed to HIV. And the "substantial amount" of both RNA and DNA found in "HIV" vesicles, Bess found, points more toward a bacterial or mycobacterial origin.

Suddenly, it seemed as if the world had been sold a bill of goods on a nonexistent retrovirus.

REFERENCES

1. Karpas A. Unusual virus produced by cultured cells from a patient with AIDS. Letter to Editor. *Mol Biol Med.* 1983; 1:457–459.
2. Karpas A, Maayan S. Lack of antibodies to adult T-cell leukemia virus and to AIDS virus in Israeli Falashas. *Nature.* 1986; 319: 794.
3. O'Hara CJ, Groopman JE. The ultrastructural and immunohistochemical demonstration of viral particles in lymph

nodes from human immunodeficiency virus-related and non-human immunodeficiency virus-related lymphadenopathy syndromes. *Hum Pathol.* 1988; 19(5): 545–549.
4. Nambuya A, Sewankambo N. Tuberculosis lymphadenitis associated with human immunodeficiency virus (HIV) in Uganda. *J Clin Pathol.* 1988; 41: 93–96.
5. Voetberg A, Lucas SB. Tuberculosis or persistent generalized lymphadenopathy in HIV disease. *Lancet.* 1991; 337: 56–57.
6. Bader JP. Reproduction of RNA humor viruses. *Comprehensive Virol.* 1975; 4: 253.
7. Gluschankof P, Mondor I. Cell membrane vesicles are a major contaminant of gradient enriched human immunodeficiency virus Type-1 preparations. *Virology.* 1997; 230(1): 125–133.
8. Bess JW. Microvesicles are a source of contaminating cellular proteins found in purified HIV-preparations. *Virology.* 1997; 230(1): 134–144.
9. Seibert FB, Feldmann FM. Morphological, biological, and immunological studies on isolates from tumors and leukemic blood. *Ann NY Acad Sci.* 1970; 174(3): 690–728.
10. Alexander-Jackson A. Specific type of microorganism isolated from animal and human cancer: bacteriology of the organism. *Growth.* 1954; 18: 37–51.
11. Livingston V. *Cancer: A New Breakthrough.* Los Angeles: Nash Publishing; 1972.
12. Cantwell AR, Jr. Histologic observation of variably acid-fast coccoid forms suggestive of cell wall deficient bacteria in Hodgkin's disease. A report of four cases. *Growth.* 1981; 45:168–187.

8/SMOKE AND MIRRORS

Like chameleons, HIV scientists continued to scurry about, changing their scientific hypotheses to blend into whatever new facts came along, much of it interpreted through the lens of earlier research done on TB and the mycobacteria. And since the doctors and scientists who bought into the HIV theory were now in the clear majority, and that majority ruled, their funding and literature mushroomed into a self-fulfilling archive such as previously had occurred with their failed HTLV-1 AIDS virus. Those who did not agree found themselves labeled "denialists" by handpicked industry attack dogs or lost their tenure or research funding, and even their jobs.

By 1983, the certain knowledge that AIDS had begun its wholesale slaughter of Africans, mainly through heterosexual sex, sent shudders down the back of a world in which not since the last great sexual pandemic of syphilis five centuries before had there been the specter of anything comparable. Men and woman were transmitting AIDS back and forth sexually in heretofore unheralded numbers.

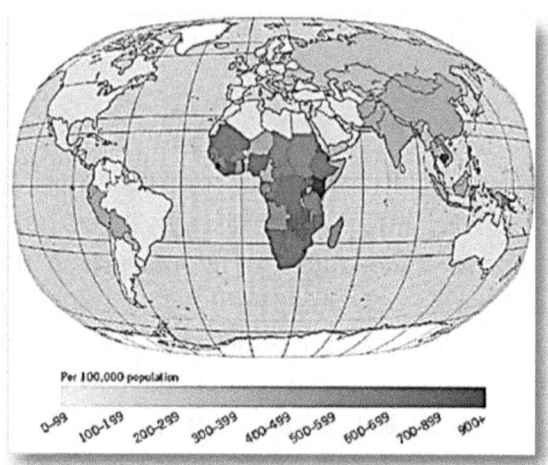

Figure 33. A Map of TB Prevalence by Country. Notice its distribution in Africa and compare to map below.

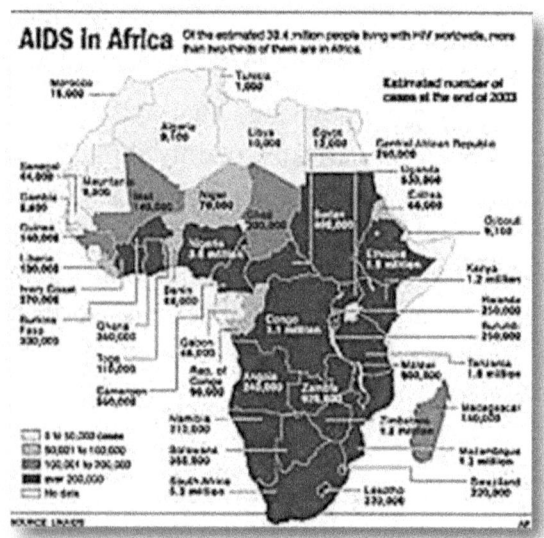

Figure 34. "AIDS" in Africa, with Roughly the Same Distribution as the TB Map above. "HIV" advocates maintain that AIDS spawns TB incidence and prevalence. Or was it the other way around?

Wave after wave of epidemic tuberculosis had hit the world. It was a disease of big numbers. It has been estimated that in the 100 years from 1850 to 1950, 1 billion persons died from tuberculosis.[1] Even today, according to the World Health Organization, TB infects over one-third of the world's inhabitants. At least one person is infected with it per second, and someone dies from TB every ten seconds. Tuberculosis, indeed, kills 2 to 3 million people each year, more than any other infectious disease in the world today. It did not need to be defined by any harmless retrovirus. It did its own defining.

From England, tuberculosis spread to the shores of Western and then Eastern Europe—and by 1900, North and South American waves began to peak. But in the developing countries of Asia and Africa, where the AIDS epidemic was still new in 1983, epidemic waves of tuberculosis had not yet reached their zenith.[2] As this TB epidemic continued to seethe, it was these very continents that would show the highest TB mortality and morbidity, even before AIDS came into the picture[3]—and would prove to be the future epicenters of AIDS.

Foreigners called the all-too-common wasting syndrome of African AIDS "slim disease." Africans themselves just called it "slim." Serwadda wrote about it in *Slim Disease: A New Disease in Uganda*,[4] but of 82 patients diagnosed with this wasting syndrome, he found 44% to have disseminated tuberculosis, earlier called "consumption," because like slim disease, TB seemed to consume the flesh off a person's skeletal structure.

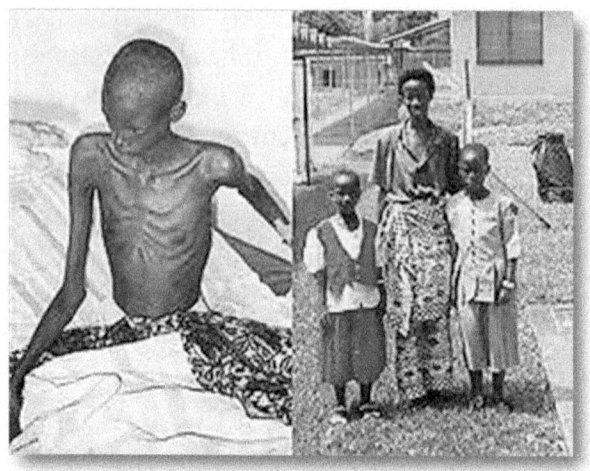

Figure 35. "Slim Disease," the Term in Uganda Used to Describe "HIV" Wasting

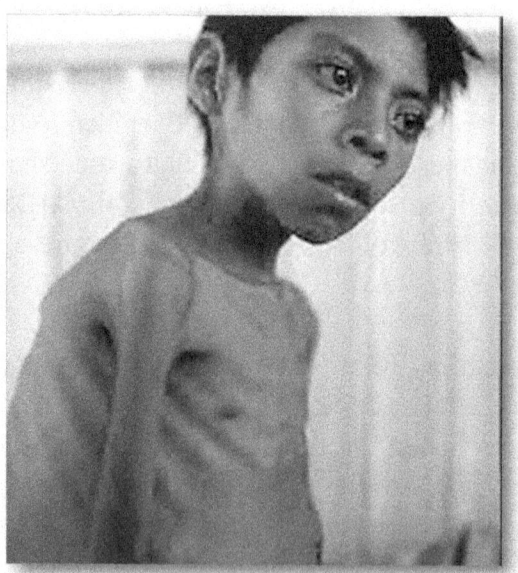

Figure 36. Tubercular "Consumption", It was known for centuries as the consuming or eating away of the flesh secondary to TB.

And so, referring to what he felt to be the tip of an iceberg, Serwadda suggested that a substantial proportion, if not all, of so-called slim disease in AIDS was actually due to disseminated tuberculosis.[5] In addition, disseminated *M. avium,* or fowl tuberculosis, was believed to be a major cause of wasting syndrome in patients with AIDS, with approximately 40% of *M. avium* victims having the same nausea or diarrhea so frequently attributed to 'HIV'.[6,7]

True, tuberculosis and diarrhea, prominent in African AIDS, had been killing Africans for some time, but suddenly they had become untreatable. Drug-resistant forms were then not so much in the public and scientific cross hairs. So a new name was needed for an old affliction. And that name, AIDS, was supplied hurriedly, perhaps too hurriedly.

It was in Africa that those who hailed HIV as the cause of AIDS faced their first and most serious challenge over extremely suspicious circumstances. Not only were over 60% of African AIDS patients not HIV-positive[8] (*Lancet*, Oct. 17, 1992), but of those who tested positive, data suggested that the antigens in HIV-1 ELISA and western blots, originally claimed to belong solely to HIV, were cross-reacting with TB and the mycobacteria.[9]

Nor was it just one but a series of "HIV" proteins that cross-reacted with tubercular proteins. Tubercular cell wall components, phenolic glycolipid (PGL), and lipoarabinomannan [LAM] were noted not only to strongly cross-react with p24, the sacred cow of 'HIV isolation', but p31, also favored in the detection of HIV in the blood.[9] Even the most prominent and persistently detected antigen in AIDS tests,[10] p41, could be found in bacteria such as tuberculosis.

Defensively, HIV diehards shot back that tuberculosis in AIDS was merely an "opportunistic infection," a label that most North American AIDS experts were originally extremely reluctant to assign. For example, to John and Kaur, in *Lancet*, the term 'opportunistic' seemed inappropriate for TB. Only infections due to normally nondisease-causing microbes should be called opportunistic.[11] *Mycobacterium tuberculosis*, the only infectious pathogen ever to force the UN to issue a (1993) global emergency, could hardly be termed nondisease-causing, according to John and Kaur, and therefore should never be labeled as opportunistic.

Many physicians were also quite wary of the contrived terms used to describe HIV. Yet they still remained silent. Makeshift expressions, like ARC (AIDS-related complex), PGL (persistent generalized lymphadenopathy) and 'pre-AIDS' were scrutinized in disbelief. There were similar forms of latent TB, yet none were ready to call them pre-tuberculosis or tuberculosis-related-complex (TRC).

By 1986, Montagnier's group, puzzled, found a patient in West Africa with AIDS but no HIV antibodies in the blood. Rather than rethink their whole hypothesis, the discoverer of HIV proceeded to simply say that it was another retrovirus at work: HIV-2, said to be responsible for a large West African epidemic, mainly transmitted through heterosexual intercourse.[12]

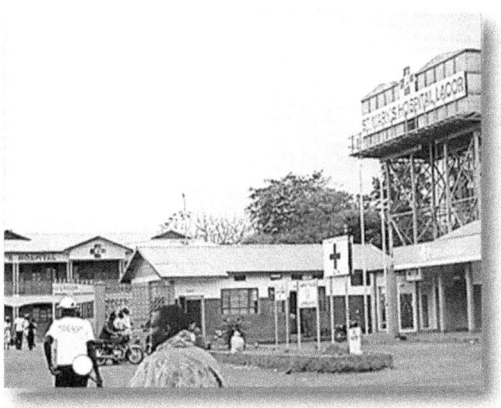

Figure 37. Lacor Hospital, Gulu, Uganda

Lacor Hospital in Gulu, Uganda, was in effect a TB sanitarium, but roughly half of the patients who remained there for two months or more came down with AIDS. And so Africans died, with the bleeding gums and anemia claimed at different times to come from both HIV and TB, but their blood was HIV-negative. In a word, they died of wasting, or consumption.

REFERENCES

1. Iseman MD. Evolution of drug resistant tuberculosis: a tale of two species. *Proc Natl Acad Sci,* USA. 1994; 91: 2428–2429.
2. Stead WW, Asim KD. Epidemiologic and host factors in tuberculosis. In: *Monographs in Infectious Disease*; vol. 2. New York: Praeger; 1983.
3. Lowell AM. *Tuberculosis in the World.* DHEW Publication No. CDC 76-8317. Washington, DC: US Government Printing Office, 1976; 3–27.

4. Serwadda D. Slim disease: a new disease in Uganda and its association with HTLV-III infection. *Lancet.* 1985; 2(8460): 849–852.
5. DeCock KM. Tuberculosis and HIV infection in sub-Saharan Africa. *JAMA.* 1992; 268: 12.
6. Kemper CA, Meng TC. Treatment of Mycobacterium avium complex bacteremia in AIDS with a four-drug oral regimen: rifampin, ethambutol, clofazimine and ciprofloxacin. *Ann Intern Med.* 1992; 116: 466–472.
7. Modilevsky T, Sattler FR. Mycobacterial disease in patients with human immunodeficiency virus infection. *Arch Intern Med.* 1989; 149: 2201–2205.
8. Hishida O, Ido E, Igarashi T, Hayami M, Miyazaki A, Ayisi NK, Osei-Kwasi M. Clinically diagnosed AIDS cases without evident association with HIV type 1 and 2 infections in Ghana. Lancet. 1992 Oct 17; 340(8825):971-2.
9. Kashala O. Infection with human immunodeficiency virus type 1 (HIV-1) and human T-cell lymphotropic viruses among leprosy patients and contacts: correlation between HIV-1 cross-reactivity and antibodies to lipoarabinomannan. *J Infect Dis.* 1994; 169(2): 296–304.
10. Veronese FM. Characterization of gp41 as the transmembrane protein coded by the HTLV-III/LAV envelope gene. *Science.* 1985; 229: 1402.
11. John JJ, Kaur A. Tuberculosis and HIV infection. *Lancet.* 1993; 342(2): 676.
12. Clavel F, Guetard D. Isolation of a new human retrovirus from West African patients with AIDS. *Science.* 1986; 233: 343–346.

9/FABRICATED SLAUGHTER

The scientific vagueness and deception to bolster the HIV theory continued. Important to the basic mechanism of AIDS is the destruction of CD4 (T-cells) lymphocytes, key to the body's resistance against infection. As this CD4 cell count falls in the blood of an AIDS patient, many treacherous infections are able to jump on board.

HIV was early on claimed to destroy these CD4 white blood cells, yet the exact mechanism for this was never made clear.[1] Papadopulos-Eleopulos points out that retroviruses were never known to kill cells. This was the one thing retrovirologists always knew and agreed on. Therefore, she asked, how could the HIV retrovirus kill CD4 cells? Instead, it seemed to Papadopulos that CD4 T-lymphocyte death might be due to the many non-HIV factors present in HIV inoculate, including other infectious agents.[2]

And although attempt after attempt has been made to say that low CD4 is synonymous with HIV, the fact is that known AIDS-risk groups may have low CD4, even in the face of persistently negative HIV antibody tests.[3,4,5]

That HIV is not the cause of apoptosis (a sort of remote-control immune cell destruction) of CD4+ cells is more than amply shown in chronically infected retroviral cell lines, where what is claimed to be "HIV" is produced, apoptosis is not detected. Even HIV discoverer Luc Montagnier (as well as others) has confirmed that HIV does not kill T-cells like CD4+ directly.[6,7]

On the other hand, virulent TB can and ferociously does depress the CD4 count,[8] and it kills T-cells like CD4+ as well as macrophages directly through nitric oxide secretion.[9]

In 1978, the first European measurement of a low CD4 in AIDS was in a patient with disseminated atypical tuberculosis (*Mycobacteria fortuitum*), closely related to *Mycobacterium tuberculosis*.[10]

As early as 1987, Canadian researchers realized that mycobacteria such as tuberculosis could alone be responsible for direct CD4 killing and much of the immunosuppression found in AIDS. Furthermore, such a tubercular immune system throttle could persist for life, even when the disease wasn't progressive.[11]

In the same vein, Mudaki, in Zaire, showed how fast a CD4 count could shrink below 200/ul just by tuberculosis, without HIV being present.[12] Moreover, TB often presented before the development of immune dysfunction, either with or without HIV.[13]

In fact, of all the infections involved in AIDS, none were associated with as low CD4 cell counts as were tubercular infections,[14] and those patients with either *M. avium* or *M. tuberculosis* in their blood had significantly lower CD4 counts.[15]

Yet there had to be more—a missing link. It has long been known that a low CD4 count in and of itself does not automatically lead to the severe immunodepression found in AIDS.[16]

REFERENCES

1. Jaworowski A, Crowe SM. Does HIV cause depletion of CD4+ T cells in vivo by the induction of apoptosis? *Immunol Cell Biol.* 1999; 77(1): 90–98.
2. Papadopulos-Eleopulos E, Turner VE. A critical analysis of the HIV-T4-Cell AIDS hypothesis. *Genetica.* 1995; 95: 5–24.
3. Detels R, English PA. Patterns of CD4+ cell changes after HIV-1 infection indicate the existence of a co-determinant of AIDS. *J Acquire Immune Defic Syndr.* 1988; 1: 390–395.
4. Donahoe RM, Bueso-Ramos C. Mechanistic implications of the findings that opiates and other drugs of abuse moderate T-cell surface receptors and antigenic markers. *Ann NY Acad Sci.* 1987; 496: 711–721.
5. Novick DM, Brown DJC. Influence of sexual preference and chronic hepatitis B virus infection on T lymphocyte subsets, natural killer activity, and suppressor. *Hepatol.* 1986; 3: 363–370.
6. Duesberg PH. AIDS acquired by drug consumption and other noncontiguous risk factors. *Pharmacol Ther.* 1992; 55: 201–277.
7. Lemaitre M, Guetard D. Protective activity of tetracycline analogs against the cytopathic effect of the human immunodeficiency viruses in CEM cells. *Res Virol.* 1990; 141(1): 5–16.
8. WHO: *Statement of AIDS and Tuberculosis.* Geneva: WHO; 1989.

9. Rojas M, Olivier M. TNF-alpha and IL-10 modulate the induction of apoptosis by virulent Mycobacterium tuberculosis in murine macrophages. *J Immunol.* 1999; 162(10): 6122–6131.
10. Bultmann BD, Flad HD. Disseminated mycobacterial histiocytosis due to M. fortuitum associated with helper T-lymphocyte immune deficiency. *Virchow's Arch.* 1982; 395: 217–225.
11. Lamoureux G, Davignon L. Is prior mycobacterial infection a common predisposing factor to AIDS in Haitians and Africans? *Ann Inst Pasteur Immunol.* 1987; 138(4): 521–529.
12. Mudaki Y, Perriens JH. Spectrum of immunodeficiency in HIV-1-infected patients with pulmonary tuberculosis in Zaire. *Lancet.* 1993; 342(8864): 143–146.
13. Reeve PA. Tuberculosis and HIV infection. *Lancet.* 1993; 342(2): 676.
14. Ohtomo K, Wang S. Secondary infections of AIDS autopsy cases in Japan with special emphasis on *Mycobacterium avium-intracellulare* complex infection. *Tohoku J Exp Med.* 2000; 192(2): 99–109.
15. Gilks CF, Richard JB. Disseminated *Mycobacterium avium* infection among HIV infected patients in Kenya. *J Acquir Immune Defic Syndr Hum Retroviral.* 1995; 8(2): 195–198.
16. John JJ, Kaur A. Tuberculosis and HIV infection. *Lancet.* 1993; 342(2): 676.

Case Western Reserve University, Ohio, July, 1998:

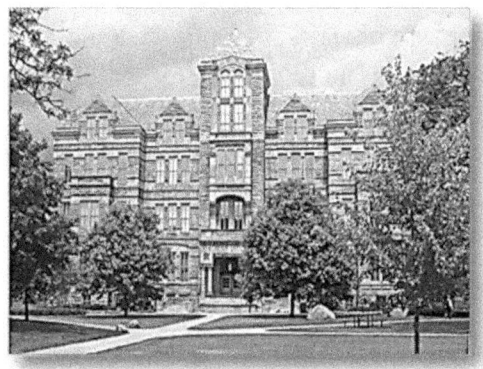

Figure 38. Case Western Reserve University, Cleveland, Ohio

Although previously demonstrated,[1,2] the actual ferocity of CD4 tubercular attack was amply shown in papers such as Hirsh's 1999 Ohio study, which showed that not only 30% of CD4 but also non-CD4 were slaughtered within 98 hours of co-culture with TB, a 20-fold increase.[3] Hirsch's electric expose was published by the *Journal of Infectious Diseases*. But it didn't stop there. The immune system's B cells[4,5] and macrophages[6,7] were also decimated by tuberculosis.

As if this wasn't enough, the fact that both TB-specific and TB-nonspecific T cells were equally affected in any tubercular attack accounted for tuberculosis's silent role in the depressed responsiveness toward such diseases as candidal thrush, pneumocystis, and other AIDS-opportunistic organisms. After all, normally it was just such nonspecific, non-CD4 lymphocytes that protected against these other diseases.

In a follow-up study, Hirsch found that destruction through apoptosis of immune cells was increased at the site of active MTB infection in patients with pleural TB, regardless of whether the patient had HIV or did not have HIV.[8] This included macrophages.

And it was the annihilation of just such infection-swallowing macrophages, critical to reticuloendothelial immune ultrastructure, that *M. tuberculosis*, *M. avium*,[9] or more certainly both working in concert, furnished the key to AIDS's comprehensive devastation of the human immune system.

REFERENCES

1. Dlugovitzky D, Luchesi S. Circulating immune complexes in patients with advanced tuberculosis and their association with autoantibodies and reduced CD4+ lymphocytes. *Braz J Med Biol Res.* 1995; 28(3): 331–335.
2. Lamoureux G, Davignon L. Is prior mycobacterial infection a common predisposing factor to AIDS in Haitians and Africans? *Ann Inst Pasteur Immunol.* 1987; 138(4): 521–529.
3. Hirsch CS, Toossi Z. Apoptosis and T-cell hyporesponsiveness in pulmonary tuberculosis. *J Infect Dis.* 1999; 179: 945–953.
4. Chaouchi N, Arvanitakis L. Characterization of transforming growth factor-B1 induced apoptosis in normal human B cells and lymphoma B cell lines. *Oncogene.* 1995; 11: 1615–1622.

5. McDonald I, Wang H. Transforming growth factor B1 cooperates with anti-immunoglobulin for the induction of apoptosis in group I (biopsy-like) Burkitt lymphoma cell lines. *Blood.* 1996; 87: 1147–1154.
6. Fratazzi C, Arbeit RD. Macrophage apoptosis in mycobacterial infections. *J Leukoc Biol.* 1999; 66(5): 763–764.
7. Molloy A, Laochumroonvorapong P. Apoptosis, but not necrosis, of infected monocytes is coupled with killing of intracellular bacillus Calmette-Guerin. *J Exp Med.* 1994; 180: 1499–1509.
8. Hirsch CS, Toossi Z, Johnson, JL, et al. Augmentation of apoptosis and interferon-γ production at sites of active *Mycobacterium tuberculosis* infection in human tuberculosis. *J of Infectious Dis.* March 1 2001; 183: 779–88.
9. Bermudez LE, Parker A. Apoptosis of Mycobacterium avium-infected macrophages is mediated by both tumour necrosis factor TNF and Fas and involves the activation of caspases. *Clin Exp Immunol.* 1999; 116: 94–99.

California Pacific Medical Center Research Institute, San Francisco, California, 1999:

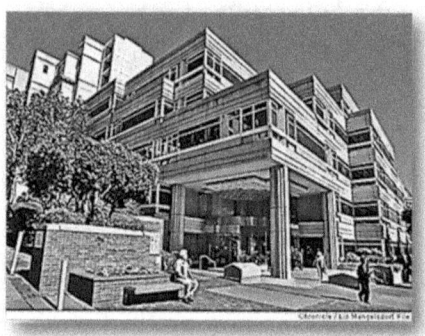

Figure 39. Part of the Pacific Campus of the California Pacific Medical Center

Conveniently, a stagnant HIV hypothesis, much in need of rejuvenation, was expanded to include infection of macrophages, long the home base of tuberculosis and now claimed to be the most important reservoir of the AIDS 'virus' from which a sustained, long-term attack on the body's lymphocytes was staged.[1] Although Duesberg and Levy saw HIV infection of macrophages as possible, neither saw their subsequent killing by HIV as a possibility.[2,3]

Indeed, key to the wanton destruction of immunity in AIDS was an attack on the macrophage. It had long been known that certain white blood cells called macrophages ate (phagocytized) bacteria, a good thing for health and well-being. And how tuberculosis and the mycobacteria became the greatest assassins ever had a lot to do with how they not only resisted lysosomal degradation once inside the macrophage, but multiplied there[4] and ate it up, from the inside out.[5] Inside every human macrophage swim two thin-membraned vacuoles: one, the phagosome, containing ingested bacteria; the other, the lysosome containing lysozyme, a destructive enzyme tailored to kill bacteria. Usually, with infection, the two fuse or join, the acidic and enzymatic content of the lysosome then killing bacterial elements harbored in the phagosome. It is how the macrophage defends the body. But after eons of evolution, virulent tubercular mycobacteria have developed a survival strategy that includes coating the phagosomes they find themselves in with proteins to prevent their enzymatic destruction,[6] punching holes into the phagosomal membrane for nutrition and the release of toxic products,[7] evading enzymatic destruction even with vacuolar fusion,[8] and learning to escape from such fused vacuoles,[9] only to eventually kill the macrophage as the hunter becomes the hunted. Thus TB and the mycobacteria enjoy and thrive in a macrophage-housed lifestyle deadly to most other pathogens.[10]

At California Pacific Research Institute, for example, Bermudez, Parker, and Petrofsky watched ferocious AIDS *M. avium* (fowl tuberculosis) destroy 28–46% more macrophages than uninfected cultures.[11] And although it was known that both *avium* and tuberculosis could escape dying macrophages only to kill and infect others, in the case of AIDS *avium*, Bermudez saw a particularly menacing event in front of him: macrophage kills only made *avium* more virulent and hungrier than ever,[12] as it sought out its next macrophage victim.

If ever therefore, an atypical virulent tuberculosis such as fowl TB could join a previous and commonly acquired latent tuberculosis with its own immune devastation, that combination would be all that was needed to create a perilous human acquired immunodeficiency. And that is exactly what the world decided to call "AIDS."

REFERENCES

1. Ho DD, Rota TR. Infection of monocyte-macrophages by human T-lymphotropic virus type III. *J Clin Invest.* 1986; 77:1712–1715.
2. Duesberg PH. AIDS epidemiology: inconsistencies with human immunodeficiency virus and with infectious disease. *Proc Natl Acad Sci.* 1991; 88: 1575–1579.
3. Levy J. Mysteries of HIV-challenges for therapy and prevention. *Nature.* 1988; 333: 519–522.
4. Armstrong JA, Hart PD. A response of cultured macrophages to *Mycobacterium tuberculosis*, with observations on fusion of lysosomes and phagosomes. *J Exp Med.* 1971; 134: 713–740.
5. Gangadharam PR, Pratt PF. In vitro response of murine alveolar and peritoneal macrophages to *Mycobacterium intracellulare*. *Am Rev Respir Dis.* 1983; 128(6): 1044–1047.
6. Pieters J. Entry and survival of pathogenic mycobacteria in macrophages. *Microbes Infect.* 2001; 3(3): 249–255.
7. Teitelbaum R, Cammer M. Mycobacterial infection of macrophages results in membrane-permeable phagosomes. *Proc Natl Acad Sci.* 1999; 96(26): 15190–15195.
8. Armstong JA, Hart PD. Phagosome–lysosome interactions in cultured macrophages infected with virulent tubercle bacilli. Reversal of the usual nonfusion pattern and observations on bacterial survival. *J Exp Med.* 1975; 142: 1–16.

9. McDonough KA, Kress Y, Bloom BR. Pathogenesis of tuberculosis: interaction of *Mycobacterium tuberculosis* with macrophages. *Infect Immun.* July 1993; 61(7): 2763–2773.
10. Rhoades ER, Ullrich HJ. How to establish a lasting relationship with your host: lessons learned from Mycobacterium spp. *Immunol Cell Biol.* 2000; 78(4): 301–310.
11. Bermudez LE, Parker A. Apoptosis of *Mycobacterium avium*-infected macrophages is mediated by both tumour necrosis factor TNF and fas and involves the activation of caspases. *Clin Exp Immunol.* 1999; 116: 94–99.
12. Bermudez LE, Parker A. Growth within macrophages increases the efficiency of *Mycobacterium avium* to invade other macrophages by complement receptor independent pathway. *Infect Immun.* 1997; 65: 1916–1925.

10/VIRAL DELUSIONS

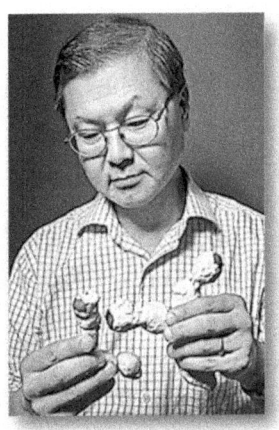

Figure 40. Dr. David Da-i Ho

By 1995, David Da-i Ho, of "It's the virus, stupid!" fame and then head of New York's Aaron Diamond AIDS Research Center, assumed the mantle of titular head of the US AIDS establishment. He and his colleagues proclaimed a new proactive stance, asserting that HIV was never inactive and multiplied astronomically in the body each day, killing CD4 cells. Ho was a Taiwanese American who pioneered the use of protease inhibitors for treating 'HIV-infected patients'.

But there was still no hard physical evidence, only theory, as to how the retrovirus called "HIV" killed. Ho speculated that the carnage took place in the lymph nodes, home of tubercular destruction for millennia, so that there were few signs of infected CD4 in the blood. Then the HIV not involved in this hypothesized slaughter shot out into the bloodstream, creating a 'viral load'. To eradicate viral load, Ho was suggesting early and aggressive antiviral drugs to be taken, probably for the life of the patient, in potent "cocktails" with serious side effects. The problem was, as Robert Gallo later noted, that just about everyone he knew realized from the start that Ho's theory was absolutely wrong.

Nevertheless, soon HIV scientists were proclaiming that the amount of virus in the blood, the so-called "viral load," was the most important determinant in AIDS prognosis.[1] But the fact is that HIV is so sparse in the blood that it requires polymerase chain reactors (PCR), a nucleic acid broth that makes copious copies of hard-to-find pathogens, to even detect it.

PCR inventor Kary Mullis would not support the use of his test to amplify and exaggerate what is being perceived as HIV in measuring 'the viral load', as is currently being done. To many, the massive amounts of RNA supposedly representing "HIV" in the circulation were suspect. Furthermore, others wanted to know, if you made a thousand copies of a dollar bill, how many real dollar bills did you actually have to begin with?

The 'viral load test', presently in use makes only copies of fragments of nucleic acids[2] attributed to HIV and does not count HIV itself. Since it does not count HIV itself, and other infections, in particular the mycobacteria such as tuberculosis, can also yield similar nucleic acid fragments, a positive viral load test cannot be regarded as signaling "HIV" itself. Meanwhile, nobody ever questioned the validity of using a non-quantitative PCR in the detection of another hard to find pathogen—tuberculosis—not even Mullis.

In 1994, British researcher John Kay walked up to a New Hampshire podium before the Proteolytic Enzyme Conference and announced that Hoffman-LaRoche's protease inhibitor RO31-8959, called saquinavir or Inverase, hadn't worked out clinically in an 18-month trial with 400 AIDS patients.³ The convenient reason given was that after an initial improvement in symptoms, HIV developed resistance to the agent, and for the time being Roche was imposing a blackout on the disappointing trial. Biochemist David Rasnick, an expert on the proteases, saw things differently. The inhibitors were performing their job as designed, which was to block HIV production. It wasn't mutation or resistance that were the problems, it was that HIV did not cause AIDS.

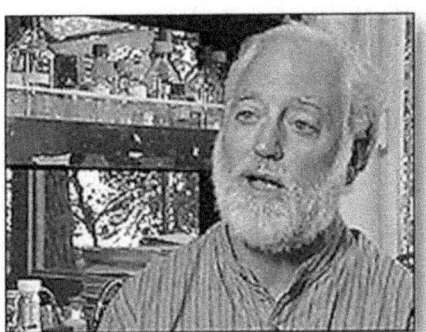

Figure 41. Dr. David Rasnick

By 1984, Rasnick was in a pivotal position to capitalize on protease momentum, but he quickly decided that to kill a harmless retrovirus was an exercise in futility, often at the risk of severe and as-yet-unknown side effects, some fatal in animals.

Although it was generally acknowledged by the HIV establishment that by the 1990s, highly active antiretroviral therapy (HAART) made headway in braking the steep rise in both AIDS and AIDS-related deaths in the United States, no randomized study to that point had ever been done comparing those who were on these drugs to those who were not.[4] Furthermore, the precipitous drop in AIDS deaths in 1995 predated by one year the introduction of the protease inhibitors, which first came onto the market in late 1996. This seems much akin to tuberculosis, which began to decrease long before any specific measures or drugs were used against it.[5]

To be sure, HAART from its onset was palliative. Specifically, with HAART, in many cases, the CD4+ count is partially restored and supposedly, therefore, the necessity for continuing drugs specifically against *M. avium* in certain cases stopped. But *M. avium* infection rebounds when these anti-HIV drugs are stopped or fail.[6] Furthermore, the antiretrovirals in HAART were not the only agents that could restore a CD4 count. This restoration also occurred in patients with HIV and TB when anti-TB treatment alone was used, as in John's study where a CD4 count of 89/ll climbed to 760/ll.[7]

In truth, the entire story of America's potent antiretroviral drugs has not nearly been unraveled. Regush mentions that the types of antiviral drugs used in the cocktails "have antimicrobial properties that could, to varying degrees, target other infections that are common to AIDS."[4] Regush was correct, and today we know that the antiretrovirals have suppressive effects on both TB and fowl tuberculosis.

FDA approval for any of these antiretroviral agents did not require information as to whether they were bactericidal, and such information is not to be found in their drug inserts. Therefore, studies that show that widespread HAART reduces the risk for TB—or may bring about the further decline of TB among persons infected with HIV—can never answer with certainty that the reason for this[8] is not some heretofore unknown direct anti-tubercular activity on the part of HAART.

For example, in 1999, Bermudez et al.[9] documented that the intense macrophage and lymphocyte killing by American AIDS *M. avium* was significantly reduced by protease inhibitors called caspases.

These investigators, in effect, established that certain protease inhibitors, a first line of defense against 'HIV' found in HAART, were able to curtail *Mycobacterium avium*'s (MAI) virulence, thus pinpointing a much more specific and satisfying reason why, all of a sudden, MAI prophylaxis was not necessary, and symptomatic improvement was noted then that HAART was "bolstering the immune system." But the questions remained: At what price in toxicity, and for how much gain in years?—an answer almost unascertainable in the face of changing definitions of what constitutes AIDS by HIV/AIDS gurus, among which was the inclusion of tuberculosis as an 'AIDS-defining' illness.

REFERENCES

1. Lyles RH, Tang AM. Virologic, immunologic, and immune activation markers as predictors of HIV-associated weight loss prior to AIDS. Multicenter AIDS cohort study. *J Acquir Immune Defic Syndr*.1999; 22(4): 386–394.

2. Johnson C. The PCR to prove HIV infection. Viral load and why they can't be used. *Continuum* (London). 1996; 4: 33–37.
3. Conlan MG. Interview with David Rasnick PhD: on Columbia's AIDS conference and the nature of science. *Zenger's News Magazine* (San Diego); 1998 Jan.
4. Regush N. *The Virus Within*. New York: Plume Press; 2001.
5. Dubos R, Dubos J. *The White Plague*. New Brunswick: Rutgers University Press; 1952.
6. Kaplan JE, Hanson MS. Epidemiology of human immunodeficiency virus-associated opportunistic infections in the United States in the era of highly active antiretroviral therapy. *Clin Infect Dis*. 2000; 30(Suppl 1): S5–S14.
7. John JJ, Kaur A. Tuberculosis and HIV infection. *Lancet*. 1993; 342(2): 676.
8. Jones JL, Hanson DL. HIV-associated tuberculosis in the era of highly active antiretroviral therapy. The adult/adolescent spectrum of HIV disease group. *Int J Tuberc Lung Dis*. 2000; 4(11): 1026–1031.
9. Bermudez LE, Parker A. Apoptosis of *Mycobacterium avium* infected macrophages is mediated by both tumor necrosis factor (TNF) and fas and involves the activation of caspases. *Clin Exp Immunol*. 1999; 116: 94–99.

11/LUCKY

Once upon a time, a small group of politically powerful scientists rammed a flawed theory on the origin and cause of AIDS down America's and then the world's throat.

Yet we are still led to believe that we are fortunate that retroviruses, only discovered in the 1970s, were uncovered just in time to label them the culprit in a killer AIDS epidemic. And lucky that two "HIVs" were discovered in rapid succession, and the technology and theory to link AIDS to the HIV retrovirus were fully in place for the first time in history, only a few years prior to the recognition of the AIDS epidemic.

Lucky? As of the 20th anniversary of the first reported AIDS case, AIDS had already infected nearly 60 million people of which almost 22 million, including nearly half a million Americans, had died, and 8,500 AIDS deaths occurred daily. Yet the prospects for a cure or vaccine are as remote as they were three decades ago.

Historically, not that long ago—at the end of the 19th century, after 150 years of denial—the medical establishment recognized that there were bacteria, and suddenly every disease seemed to be caused by bacteria. But with the advent of the electron microscope, unknown disease was more and more attributed to a virus or a retrovirus, often to no avail. Thus it was that scientists were certain that a virus was behind Lyme disease, mycoplasma pneumonia, and Legionnaires' disease before their respective bacteria were found.

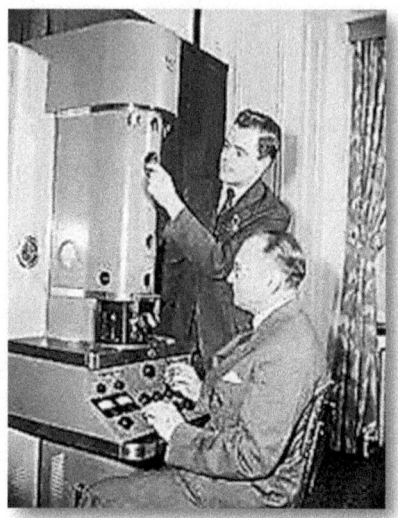

Figure 42. Vladimir Zworykin (seated) and James Hillier Demonstrate an Early Electron Microscope.

By 1931, Rudenberg, hoping to visualize the polio virus, filed a patent for his electron microscope, and during WWII investigators never gave up on an electron search for a cancer retrovirus, despite one dismal failure after another.

Then an AIDS "virus" was found, primarily because it was looked for, and not because it caused AIDS—and was soon bolstered by half-truths, flawed theory, and downright hocus-pocus.

HIV scientists said that "unassailable" epidemiological evidence[1] established HIV or a virus as the cause of AIDS, including those epidemiological studies carried out by the CDC on filtered factor VIII blood transfusions for hemophiliacs. Blattner cites Peterman in his article[2] as saying, "It is also noteworthy that HIV infection, and not infection with any other infectious agent, is linked to blood transfusion-associated AIDS." But blood transfusions do not distinguish between HIV and other filterable infectious agents especially, as in the case of tubercular mycobacteria, if these other infectious agents are not screened for. Yet one of the original factor VIII transfusion cases happened in Canton, Ohio, yielding a diagnosis of oral thrush and disseminated *Mycobacterium avium*.[3]

John Lattimer could not foresee the unusual situation that, decades later, might be involved with the direct insemination of particularly virulent tubercular mycobacteria rectally onto the vulnerable one-layered epithelium of the prostate during gay sex. Nor could Lattimer forecast the hypervirulent strains of AIDS *M. tuberculosis* and *M. avium* that would one day, decades later, be shared in much greater numbers heterosexually in a worldwide epidemic called AIDS. But who could have? Nor could Gondzik realize the profound significance of warning his patients, on the eve of the AIDS epidemic in 1979, to wear condoms lest they acquire sexually transmitted tuberculosis.[4]

Mycobacterial infections are the main cause of bacterial infection during AIDS[5] and often precede other infections by one to ten months.[6] The fact that three decades after AIDS started killing people, tubercular mycobacteria, despite their prevalence in AIDS, are not considered its cause is in no small part due to the inability of scientists and the lay public to understand the ability of mycobacterial and tubercular infection, once contracted, to lie seemingly dormant for extended lengths of time in humans[7] and at the same time begin to melt the immune system away.[8]

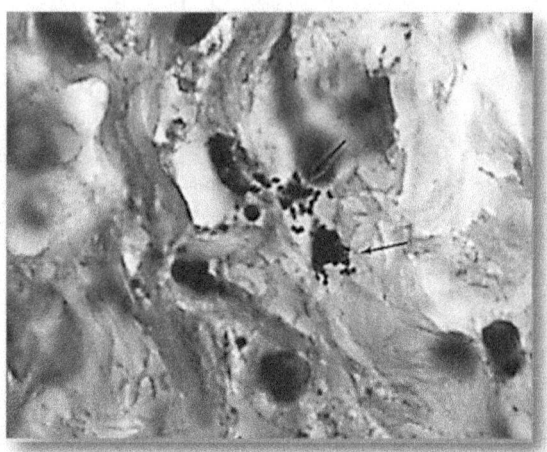

Figure 43. Tissue Section of Lung in Fatal AIDS. Arrows point to round tubercular forms. These forms cultured out from bronchoscopic washings as *Mycobacterium avium* or fowl tuberculosis (below), acid-fast stain, X1000 in oil.

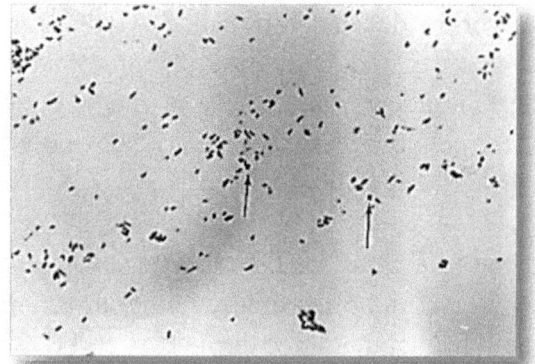

Figure 44. Lab culture of Fowl tuberculosis [Mycobacterium avium] Cultured from the Patient Above. The culture is pleomorphic (has many forms), both acid-fast and not acid-fast. These vary in size. Acid-fast stain X1000, in oil.

Nor was it emphasized that both tuberculosis, whose chronic lymphadenitis (lymph node inflammation) is its most common extrapulmonary (outside the lung) manifestation,[9] and *M. avium*, the most common cause of lymphadenitis in children,[10] can attack lymph nodes[11] and the entire body additively and simultaneously.[12]

AIDS is a mycobacterial disease, and patients with advanced TB or avium are indistinguishable from those with 'HIV'. Even in the earliest AIDS cases on record, dating back to 1959, tuberculosis[13] and the atypical mycobacteria[14,15] were clinically and bacteriologically diagnosed.

Perhaps one of the most convincing arguments for the intimate causal link between tubercular infection and AIDS comes from the widespread geographical overlap of the two. Worldwide, by the most conservative estimates, around one in three people is infected with *Mycobacteria tuberculosis* alone, or 1.8 billion people,[16] and the very cities in which up to 80% have tuberculosis are the epicenters of AIDS. The last world AIDS conference, which was held in Barcelona, admitted that a third of all AIDS deaths were from diagnosed tuberculosis.[17]

Almost a million new cases of AIDS were estimated to be attributable to tuberculosis in 1995, and by the year 2000 there were probably 8 million co- infected individuals worldwide.[18] Figures such as these make it unconvincing that AIDS ever surpassed tuberculosis as the leading cause of death in the world, especially in lieu of cross-reacting sera, which opens up the question as to just how many cases attributed to HIV are in fact from tuberculosis or its allied mycobacteria.

Dual Pathogen Concept

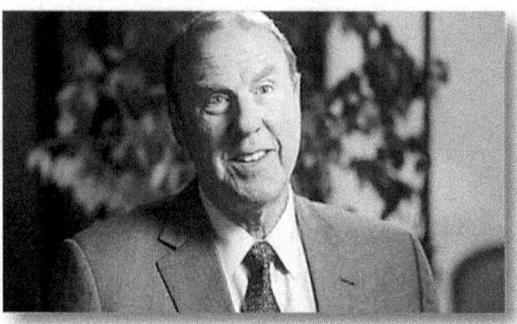

Figure 45. Dr. Michael Gottlieb: Immunologist and Associate Clinical Professor of Medicine, the David Geffen School of Medicine, UCLA, Los Angeles.

When the AIDS epidemic officially began in June 1981, allergist-immunologist Michael Gottlieb of UCLA, after first implicating cytomegalovirus (CMV), said in a headline, *"Ongoing AIDS Epidemic Could Be Product of Dual Pathogen Infection,"* concluding that AIDS resulted from not one but two microbial infections.[19] This theory presented an interesting possibility not specifically addressed by Gottlieb. Unexpected in early AIDS autopsies was the surprisingly high proportion of difficult-to-diagnose fowl tuberculosis, or *Mycobacterium avium-intracellulare*,[20] in up to 55% of American cases.[21] But in Haitian and African AIDS patients, undoubtedly just as exposed to *avium*, death by *Mycobacterium tuberculosis* predominated. Gottlieb had himself referred several AIDS patients with fowl tuberculosis or *avium* to Zakowski for further study at the UCLA Medical Center.

Indeed, most convincing evidence points to Gottlieb's proposed dual pathogen thoughts as in reality being atypical mycobacteria such as *avium* somehow getting into a human blood pool already harboring latent or active *M. tuberculosis*. The "acquired" in acquired immunodeficiency syndrome is *M. avium* or a similar non-tuberculous mycobacteria; "immune deficiency" is but the result of a savage double attack on the immune system by an atypical mycobacterium (such as *M. avium*) and *M. tuberculosis*. *Avium* alone has, in the short space of 30 years, gone from relative obscurity to the leading infectious disease in US and European AIDS, And there is no dearth of literature to explain just how this could have happened—ranging from human sexual transmission,[22,23] to bestiality,[22,24] to certain Voodoo practices such as African ritualistic drinking of animal blood,[25] to the medical or addicts' use of shared needles.[26] Thus was the groundwork laid for a combined tubercular and mycobacterial mayhem—the introduction and spread of virulent atypical mycobacteria into the human blood pool, whether in Africa, the United States, Europe, or the rest of the world.

From the onset, lymph nodes were recognized to be important in AIDS. And if in the late 1960s, lymph nodes from 368 swine from Transvaal and Natal, South Africa, were examined and found to mostly contain *M. avium complex* (MAC),[27] these very same tubercular strains reappeared—as smoking guns—in the lymph nodes of African AIDS victims in the early 1970s.[28]

Only a few strains of MAC (*M. avium complex*) are found in human AIDS.[29] Notably, these are also found in the simian AIDS in monkeys.[30] Weiszfeiler and Karczag[31] succeeded in isolating 50 strains of mycobacteria, including MAC from monkeys[32]— significant in that millions of pre-AIDS Africans were vaccinated with an early polio vaccine attenuated in living monkey kidney tissue. Some saw a correlation between where the bulk of polio vaccine was administered and the epicenters of AIDS.[33] The *simian-avium* (SAV) group of mycobacteria share characteristics of both *Mycobacterium avium* and *Mycobacterium simiae*, which by itself is entirely capable of causing a lethal AIDS infection.[34] Also soil-borne MAC is found in cats, swine, and primates, all significant in early retroviral theories regarding AIDS.

The fertile soil upon which *M. avium* and similar "atypical" mycobacteria plants AIDS is preexisting TB, often latent, always immunosuppressive. Despite WHO estimates, Fox maintained that nearly half the world has TB,[35] but others feel that number to be even greater.

Cantwell, who repeatedly found tubercular acid-fast forms in AIDS, felt it reasonable to assume that the initial immunosuppression in that disease must also be present in many "healthy" people, as studies indicate that some promiscuous but otherwise healthy gays were actually immunosuppressed to begin with.[36] *Mycobacteria tuberculosis*, both with its vast reservoir of seemingly well and its human immune-killing potential, certainly fulfills this criterion. Papadopulos-Eleopulos[37] mentions that in African AIDS, HIV infection usually follows TB.

The first case of human disease due to *M. avium-intracellulare* (MAC) was reported in a middle-aged Mesabi Range iron miner in 1943. His symptoms were pulmonary,[38] and until the emergence of AIDS, lung infection alone typified *avium*, though differentiation between fowl or *avium* tuberculosis and tuberculosis itself was at times nearly impossible.[39] The first reports of MAC in AIDS appeared in 1982, where Zakowski found that "all of the homosexual patients that have died of acquired immunodeficiency at the UCLA Medical Center for the Health Sciences have had disseminated MAC infection."[40] Furthermore, the team mentions, "Because of this preliminary observation, we now vigorously seek evidence of mycobacterial infection in homosexuals with unexplained lymphadenopathy."

Soon the devastatingly immunosuppressive potential of co-infection with *M. tuberculosis* and *M. avium* was shown.[12] As already mentioned, this ability of mycobacteria to attack simultaneously is a recurrent theme in the literature. But in AIDS, it would bring on a combined immunosuppression the likes of which man had never had to deal with. The documented ability for AIDS and TB to potentiate one another[41] is a result of such a double-pronged mycobacterial attack between AIDS, the atypical tubercular mycobacterial infection—and tuberculosis.

In such a scenario, "HIV" is simply one of the L-forms of an atypical tuberculosis, in particular *M. avium*, and until it is recognized as such, no 'retroviral' vaccine or cure will be possible, because it is not a retrovirus that is causing AIDS.

In the United States, on the surface, AIDS is characterized by the severe immunosuppression of *M. avium* [MAC] and opportunistic infections like Kaposi's sarcoma and *Pneumocystis carinii*. In Africa, it is a wasting disease characteristically ending with death by *Mycobacteria tuberculosis*. The human immunodeficiency virus should cause the same disease, were it from the same cause.

In disseminated *Mycobacterium avium* infection among HIV-infected patients in Kenya, Gilks approaches this most perplexing AIDS enigma in terms of the mycobacteria, addressing the apparent relative rarity of disseminated MAC in AIDS in Africa and the developing countries.[42] That MAC exists in the African as well as the American environment[43] cannot be denied. Nor can the fact that African skin tests prove antibodies to MAC are already in African blood.[44] Gilks acknowledges that AIDS patients in developing countries are probably dying of more virulent tubercular infections before they become immunosuppressed enough to show *avium*. Inderlied[45] and O'Keefe[46] agree. Therefore, it is not that an atypical mycobacteria like *avium* is not present in concert with TB at the beginning of the severe immunosuppression called AIDS, it is that it is not often being picked up early in the disease, because the extent of immunosuppression has not been achieved for *avium* to become obvious.

Gilks[42] mentions that AIDS patients in Africa, already infected with latent tuberculosis, are more likely to reactivate this mycobacteria with catastrophic results before reaching the low CD4 level associated with clinical MAC. This, however, does not preclude the fact that *avium* or similar non-tubercular mycobacteria, as causative, plants AIDS in the soil of previous tubercular infection, whether in Africa or elsewhere.

The full extent of drug-resistant TB in African countries is unknown but at least as prevalent as it is in New York, Haiti, or the Ivory Coast.[47] Frieden found 30% of resistant strains of tuberculosis in New York AIDS patients,[48] but Shafer assured that with or without HIV, drug-resistant tuberculosis was comparable.[49] How much of multidrug-resistant (MDR) TB is in fact a fusion with the atypical mycobacteria like MAC or SAV is an open question. Meanwhile, there hasn't been a new TB drug in 37 years.[50] And for its part, *avium* (swine or fowl tuberculosis) and the 'atypical' mycobacteria in man has never had a truly satisfactory treatment.[51] Whether this situation will change with novel strategies now in the pipeline remains to be seen.[52]

It is only fitting that a bizarre tale—the history and promotion of HIV and its drug cocktails—ends in a bizarre way: that the only real benefit of the drugs called antiretrovirals is to try to contain tubercular infections in a fairly toxic manner, which they were not designed to do in the first place.

Yet until some honest reassessment of the situation occurs among the reactionary and monetary forces that have handed us this, millions will be the slaves to substandard, at times toxic treatment using antiretrovirals for a disease that is of mycobacterial origin and causation to begin with.

REFERENCES

1. Blattner W, Gallo RC. HIV causes AIDS. *Science*. 1988; 241(4865): 515–516.
2. Peterman TA, Stoneburner RL. Risk of human immunodeficiency virus transmission from heterosexual adults with transfusion-associated infections. *JAMA*. 1988; 259: 53.
3. Elliot JL, Hoppes WL. The acquired immunodeficiency syndrome and *Mycobacterium avium-intracellulare* in a patient with hemophilia. *Ann Intern Med*. 1983; 98: 290–293.

4. Gondzik M, Jasiewicz J. Experimental study on the possibility of tuberculosis transmission by coitus. *Z Urol Nphrol.* 1979; 72(12): 911–914.
5. Perrone C. Mycobacterial infections in AIDS. *Rev Prat.* 1995; 45(6): 729–732.
6. Bisburg E. Central nervous system tuberculosis with the acquired immunodeficiency syndrome and its related complex. *Ann Intern Med.* 1986; 105: 210–213.
7. Youmans GP. In: *Tuberculosis.* Philadelphia: WB Saunders; 1979:318–325.
8. Lamoureux G, Davignon L. Is prior mycobacterial infection a common predisposing factor to AIDS in Haitians and Africans? *Ann Inst Pasteur Immunol.* 1987; 138(4): 521–529.
9. Jawahar MS. Scrofula revisited: an update on the diagnosis and management of tuberculosis of superficial lymph nodes. *Indian J Pediatr.* 2000; 67(2): 528–533.
10. Hazra R, Robson CD. Lymphadenitis due to nontuberculous mycobacteria in children: presentation and response to therapy. *Clin Infect Dis.* 1999; 28(1): 123–129.
11. Terrones R, de Alarcon A. Mixed adenitis caused by *Mycobacterium avium complex* and *Mycobacterium tuberculosis complex* in patients with HIV infection. *Enferm Infect Microbiol Clin.* 1997; 15(4): 225–226.
12. Tsukamura M, Mizuno S. Occurrence of *Mycobacterium tuberculosis* and strains of the *Mycobacterium avium–M. intracellulare complex* together in the sputum of patients with pulmonary tuberculosis. *Tubercle.* 1981; 62: 43–46.
13. Williams G, Stretton TB, Leonard JC. AIDS in 1959? *Lancet.* 1983; 2: 1136.

14. Hagmar B, Kutti J. Disseminated infection caused by *Mycobacterium kansasii*. Report of a case and brief review of the literature. *Acta Med Scand.* 1969; 186: 93–99.
15. Schonell ME, Crofton JW. Disseminated infection with *Mycobacterium avium*. *Tubercle.* 1968; 49: 12–30.
16. World Health Organization (WHO). *WHO Report on the Tuberculosis Epidemic, 1995*. Geneva: World Health Organization; 1995.
17. Naik G. Agency to unveil a joint assault on TB and HIV. *Wall Street J.* July 9, 2002.
18. Quinn TC. HIV–AIDS-related problems in developing countries from HIV and AIDS, In: *Infectious Diseases* by Armstrong and Cohen. London: Mosby-Wolfe; 1999.
19. Gottlieb MS. Ongoing AIDS epidemic could be product of dual pathogen infection. *Skin and Allergy News.* 1983; 14.
20. Welch K., Finkbeiner W. Autopsy findings in the acquired immune deficiency syndrome. *JAMA.* 1984; 252: 1152–1159.
21. Kiehn TE, Edwards FF. Infections caused by *Mycobacterium avium complex* in immunocompromised patients: diagnosis by blood culture and fecal examination, antimicrobial susceptibility tests, and morphological and seroagglutination characteristics. *J Clin Microbiol.* 1985; 21: 168–173.
22. Damsker B, Bottone EJ. *Mycobacterium avium–Mycobacterium intracellulare* from the intestinal tracts of patients with the acquired immunodeficiency syndrome: concepts regarding acquisition and pathogenesis. *J Infect Dis.* 1985; 151(1): 179–181.
23. DeCaprariis PJ, Giron JA. *Mycobacterium avium-intracellulare* infection and possible venereal transmission. *Ann Intern Med.* 1984; 101(5): 721.

24. Katner HP. Origin of AIDS. *J Natl Med Assoc.* 1988; 80: 262.
25. Rapoza N. An AIDS expert's grim message. *Am Med News.* December 5, 1986.
26. Roberts DJ. *Tuberculosis and HIV Infection in Africa.* 1989; 298(1): 751.
27. Kleeberg HH, Nel EE. Porcine mycobacterial lymphadenitis. *J S Afr Vet Med Assoc.* 1969; 40: 233–250.
28. Kleeberg HH, Gartig D. Experience with sample surveys among African tribes and their annual risk of infection. In: *23rd International Tuberculosis Conference*, Mexico City, Sept 22–26, 1975.
29. Kiehn TE, Edwards FF. Infections caused by *Mycobacterium avium complex* in immunocompromised patients: diagnosis by blood culture and fecal examination, antimicrobial susceptibility tests, and morphological and seroagglutination characteristics. *J Clin Microbiol.* 1985; 21: 168–173.
30. Henrickson RV, Maul DH. Epidemic of acquired immunodeficiency in rhesus monkeys. *Lancet.* 1983; 1: 388–390.
31. Weiszfeiler JG, Karczag E. Study of mycobacteria strains belonging to the avian-intracellular group isolated from monkeys. *Ann Soc Beig Med Trop.* 1973; 53(4): 315–320.
32. Papadopulos-Eleopulos E, Turner VF. AIDS in Africa: distinguishing fact and fiction. *World J Microbiol Biotechnol.* 1995; 11: 135–143.
33. Hooper E. *The River: A Journey to the Source of HIV and AIDS.* Boston: Little Brown and Company; 1999.
34. MMWR Disseminated infection with simiae-avium group mycobacteria in persons with AIDS—Thailand and Malawi, 1997. *Centers for Disease Control and Prevention (CDC).* 2002; 51(23): 501–2.

35. Fox JL. TB: A grim disease of numbers. *ASM News.* 1990; 56: 363–364.
36. Cantwell AR, Jr. *AIDS: The Mystery and the Solution.* Los Angeles: Aries Rising Press; 1983.
37. Papadopulos-Eleopulos E, Turner VF. AIDS in Africa: distinguishing fact and fiction. *World J Microbiol Biotechnol.* 1995; 11: 135–143.
38. Feldman WH, Davies HE. An unusual mycobacterium isolate from sputum of a man suffering from pulmonary disease of long duration. *Am Rev Tuberc.* 1943; 48: 272–290.
39. Ortbals DW, Marr JJ. A comparative study of tuberculosis and other mycobacterial infections and their associations with malignancy. *Am Rev Respir Dis.* 1978; 117: 39–45.
40. Zakowski P, Fligiel S. Disseminated *Mycobacterium avium-intracellulare* infection in homosexual men dying of acquired immunodeficiency. *JAMA.* 1982; 248: 2980–2982.
41. Goldman KP. AIDS and tuberculosis. *Br Med J.* 1987; 295: 511–512.
42. Gilks CF, Richard JB. Disseminated *Mycobacterium avium* infection among HIV infected patients in Kenya. *J Acquir Immune Defic Syndr Hum Retroviral.* 1995; 8(2): 195–198.
43. Von Reyn CF, Waddel RD. Isolation of *Mycobacterium avium complex* from water in the United States, England, Zaire, and Kenya. *J Clin Microbiol.* 1993a; 31: 3227–3230.
44. Von Reyn CF, Barber TW. Evidence of previous infection with *M. avium* among healthy subjects: an international study of dominant mycobacterial skin test reactions. *J Infect Dis.* 1993b; 168: 1553–1558.
45. Inderlied CB, Kemper CA. The *Mycobacterium avium complex. Clin Microbiol Rev.* 1993: 266–310.

46. O'Keefe EA, Wood R. AIDS in Africa. *Scand J Gastroenterol Suppl.* 1996; 220: 147–152.
47. Long R. Impact of human immunodeficiency virus type 1 on tuberculosis in rural. *Haiti Am Rev Respir Dis.* 1991; 143: 69–73.
48. Frieden TR, Sterling T. The emergence of drug-resistant tuberculosis in New York City. *New Engl J Med.* 1993; 328: 521–526.
49. Shafer RW, Chirgwin KD. HIV prevalence, immunosuppression and drug resistance in patients with tuberculosis in an area endemic for AIDS. *AIDS.* 1991; 5: 399–405.
50. Naik G. Agency to unveil a joint assault on TB and HIV. *Wall Street J.* July 9, 2002.
51. Hafner R, Inderlied DM. Correlation of quantitative bone marrow and blood cultures in AIDS patients with disseminated *Mycobacterium avium complex* infection. *J Infect Dis.* 1999; 180: 438–447.
52. Broxmeyer L, Sosnowska D, Miltner E, Chacon O, Wagner D, McGarvey J, et al. Killing of *Mycobacterium avium* and *Mycobacterium tuberculosis* by a mycobacteriophage delivered by a nonvirulent mycobacterium: a model for phage therapy of intracellular bacterial pathogens. *J Infect Dis.* 2002; 186.

ABOUT THE AUTHOR

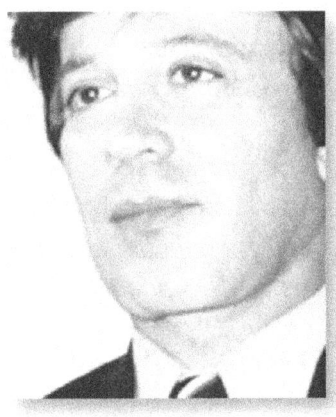

Lawrence Broxmeyer, MD, is a Pennsylvania internist/medical researcher. He was on staff at New York affiliate hospitals of SUNY Downstate, Cornell University, and New York University for approximately fourteen years, part of which was during the height of the US Coastal AIDS epidemic. In conjunction with colleagues in San Francisco and at the University of Nebraska, he pursued, as lead author and originator, a novel technique to kill AIDS mycobacteria and tuberculosis, producing outstanding results (see *Journal of Infectious Diseases* October 15, 2002; 186(8): 1155–60). His ideas on killing intracellular pathogens by phage have influenced and stimulated further research in this area to this day. Recently he contributed a chapter regarding these findings to Sleator and Hill's textbook *Patho-Biotechnology*, published by Landes Bioscience. In addition, Broxmeyer has written many peer-reviewed articles, available on PubMed of the US Library of Medicine, National Institutes of Health, at: http://www.ncbi.nlm.nih.gov/pubmed?term=broxmeyer%20L. Broxmeyer's research covers the most challenging medical problems of our times, including AIDS, Alzheimer's disease, diabetes, Parkinson's, and cardiovascular disease. Among the books that Dr. Broxmeyer has published is *Parkinson's— Another Look*, by New Century Press, in its 3rd edition. ISBN-13: 978-1890035266.

Excerpts from reviews of Broxmeyer's AIDS book are below:
"I am of the opinion that this book may offer a solution to the mystery surrounding the AIDS pandemic with regard to a possible vaccine or cure for AIDS in the near future.
Finally, the author should be congratulated for "daring where angels fear to tread."
—Professor PS Igbigbi

"I have never learned so much in such a short time—your book AIDS: What the Discoverers of HIV Have Never Admitted, *is absolutely the most revealing and clearly documented work I've ever read! Talk about a superb journalistic documentary—amazing."*
—Douglass Alexander, PhD

"I think you are a pioneer...you have to make the discoveries because apparently no one has gone there before you! Sometimes the best beginning discoveries are the people who ask the controversial questions that cast doubt on the status quo. Like WHAT IF?"
—Alan Cantwell Jr., MD

AIDS Book Review Journal
University of Illinois at Chicago
H. Robert Malinowsky, Editor
ISSN 1068-4174
Number 71

"*An interesting book that presents the hypothesis that AIDS may be caused by a strain of tuberculosis, which would mean that tuberculosis and atypical tuberculosis are not opportunistic diseases but actually triggers for becoming HIV positive, which results in AIDS. Interesting reading. It has extensive references. For those doing research, this would be a curious little book to read.*"

INDEX

A

Actinomycin D, 35
Africa, 81–82, 85, 116
African swine flu virus, 28
AIDS
   in Africa, 81–82, 85
   causes of, 3–4
   dual-pathogen theory of, 112–113
   female to male transmission of, 49
   high-risk populations for, 24
   history of, 21–26
   infectious deaths in, 15, 17
   mortality rates for, 107
   as mycobacterial disease, 111
   sexual transmission of, 23, 49
   statistics regarding, 3, 107
   tubercular infection and, 111
AIDS-defining illnesses, 8, 13, 105
AIDS-related complex, 86
Alexander-Jackson, Eleanor, 44, 46, 71
Antiretrovirals
   antibiotic effect and, 6
   CD4 counts affected by, 6
   facial lipoatrophy caused by, 11–12
   fowl tuberculosis affected by, 6
   lifespan affected by, 5, 11
   palliative use of, 104
   toxicity of, 11
   tuberculosis affected by, 6, 117
Apoptosis, of CD4+ cells, 89–90
Armed Forces Institute of Pathology, 41
ASFV. *See* African swine flu virus
Atherosclerosis, 11
Atypical tuberculosis
   cell-wall-deficient, 16–17, 42
   Montagnier's studies, 42

B

B cells, 93

Bacteria
  L-forms of, 37–38, 45, 71, 79, 115
  mycobacteria. *See* Mycobacteria
Barré-Sinoussi, Françoise, 12, 14–15, 69–70, 73–74
Bestiality, 65

C
California Pacific Medical Center, 96–97
Cambridge University Clinical School, 77
Case Western Reserve University, 93
Caspases, 105
Cat leukemia, 26–27
CD4+ cells
  antiretrovirals effect on, 6, 104
  antitubercular therapies effect on, 104
  apoptosis of, 89–90
  description of, 25
  HIV destruction of, 89
  tuberculosis effects on, 90, 93
CDC, 2
Cell-wall-deficient atypical tuberculosis, 16–17, 42
Cell-wall-deficient bacteria, 37–38
Centre on HIV/AIDS, 9

Children
  lymph node involvement in, 15
  lymphadenitis in, 111
Chronic lymphadenitis, 111
"Consumption," 83–84, 87
Coronary artery disease, 11
Curran, James, 25
Cytomegalovirus, 25, 112

D
Damsker, Beca, 64–66
De Caprariis, Pascal, 62
Dowdle, Walter, 30
Doxycycline, 42
Drug addicts, 24
Drug-resistant tuberculosis, 116
Duesberg, Peter, 75
Dugas, Gaëtan, 4, 23

E
Electron microscope, 107–108
ELISA screening test, 9–10
Essex, Myron "Max," 9–10, 27–28, 30

F
Facial lipoatrophy, 11–12
Feline leukemic virus (FeLV), 27–28
Female to male transmission, 49
Fowl tuberculosis. *See also* *Mycobacterium avium*

as AIDS-defining illnesses, 8, 13, 66, 112
antiretrovirals effect on, 6
in cats, 29
characteristics of, 65
Damsker's findings, 64
histology of, 110
incidence of, 7
lymph node involvement by, 14, 113
macrophages affected by, 97
sexual transmission of, 62
in United States, 12–13
wasting syndrome caused by, 85
Francis, Donald, 25–26

G
Gallo, Robert, 25, 27, 45–46, 74–75, 78, 102
"Gay-related immune deficiency," 22
Genital tuberculosis, 54
Genital Tuberculosis, a Forgotten Disease?, 57
Gottlieb, Michael, 112

H
HAART. *See* Highly active antiretroviral therapy
Hardy, William, 27
Hemophiliacs, 24

Highly active antiretroviral therapy, 5–6, 104–105
High-risk populations, 24
Hillier, James, 108
HIV
  CDC estimates of, 2
  discovery of, 108–109
  ELISA screening test for, 9–10
  Ho's hypotheses about, 101–102
  new cases of, 2
  tuberculosis and, 8, 111, 114
HIV-2, 86
Ho, David Da-i, 3, 101
Homosexuals, 12, 21
HTLV. *See* Human leukemic retrovirus
HTLV-1, 28–30, 69, 73, 77, 81
HTLV-2, 28
HTLV-3, 74
Human growth hormone, 46
Human leukemic retrovirus, 30
Hypothesis on the Origin of Genital Tuberculosis in the Two Sexes, 57

I
Institute of Human Virology, 9

J
Jarrett, William, 27
Jarrett virus leukemia, 27

Journal of Infectious Diseases,
   4, 65, 93
Journal of the American Medical Association, 15

K
Kaposi's sarcoma, 22–25, 115
Karpas, Abraham, 77–78
Kashala, Oscar, 9–10
Kay, John, 103
Kinshasa University Medical School, 10
Klieneberger, Emy, 37–38
Koch, Robert, 29

L
Laboratory of Viral Diagnostics, 9
Lacor Hospital, 87
Lancet, 86
Latent tuberculosis, 116
Lattimer, John K., 52–53, 55–56, 109
LAV. *See* Lymphadenopathy-associated virus
Lentivirus, 74–75
L-forms, 37–38, 45, 71, 79, 115
Lifespan, highly active antiretroviral therapy effects on, 5, 11
Lipoarabinomannan, 85

Livingston, Virginia, 35–36, 42, 45–46, 76, 79
Lo, Shyh-Ching, 41–42
Lymph nodes
   fowl tuberculosis involvement of, 14, 113
   Montagnier's studies of, 70–71
   tuberculosis involvement of, 14, 30
Lymphadenitis, chronic, 111
Lymphadenopathy, 13
Lymphadenopathy-associated virus, 69–70, 76

M
Macrophages, 93–94, 96–97
Manhattan, 21–26
Metabolic syndrome, 11
Minocycline, 42
Montagnier, Luc, 4, 12, 25, 30, 38, 42, 69–71, 73–74, 78, 90
Mount Sinai Hospital, 64–66
MTB infection, 94
Much, Hans, 71
Much's granules, 71
Mullis, Kary, 15, 102
Multidrug-resistant tuberculosis, 117
Mycobacteria

bacterial infections caused by, 109
CD4+ cells affected by, 90
description of, 38
sexual transmission of, 55
simian-avium group of, 114, 117
tubercular, 109–110. *See also* Tuberculosis
Mycobacteria smegmatis, 55
Mycobacterium avium, 9. *See also* Fowl tuberculosis
in AIDS patients, 58, 113, 116
antiretrovirals effect on, 6
in blood products, 109
CD4 cell counts affected by, 90
deaths caused by, 17
disseminated, 116
filterable forms of, 71
histology of, 13, 110
macrophages affected by, 94, 97
Mycobacterium tuberculosis and, co-infection of, 115
protease inhibitors effect on, 105
wasting syndrome caused by, 85

Mycobacterium avium complex, 113
Mycobacterium avium-intracellulare
in AIDS patients, 115
characteristics of, 65
description of, 7
human disease caused by, 114
sexual transmission of, 58, 62, 65
Mycobacterium tuberculosis
in AIDS patients, 112
CD4 cell counts affected by, 90
deaths caused by, 17, 112
genital transmission of, 50, 55
global prevalence of, 111
latent infections of, 12
macrophages affected by, 94
Mycobacterium avium and, co-infection of, 115
as opportunistic infection, 86

N
National Cancer Act, 36
National Cancer Institute, 74
National Cancer Program, 36

National Institute of Allergy and Infectious Diseases, 2, 7
National Serology Reference Laboratory, 9
Neck lymphadenopathy, 13
Niagara Peninsula Sanatorium, 54
NIAID. *See* National Institute of Allergy and Infectious Diseases
Nixon, Richard, 36

O
Opportunistic infections
   Curran's theory on, 25
   description of, 17
   Kaposi's sarcoma, 22–25, 115
   Pneumocystis carinii, 22, 115

P
p24, 85
p41, 86
Pasteur Institute, 69–71, 73
Patient Zero, 23
Peer, Edgar T., 54–55
Penile ulcers
   HIV and, 57
   tuberculosis as cause of, 56, 58
Peripheral artery disease, 11
Persistent generalized lymphadenopathy, 86

Perth Group, 16
Pharmaceutical companies, 6–7
Phenolic glycolipid, 85
Pneumocystis carinii, 22, 115
Polymerase chain reaction, 49
"Pre-AIDS," 86
Prostatic tuberculosis, 52–53
Prostatitis, 49
Protease inhibitors, 101, 103

Q
Queens Hospital Center, 62

R
Rasnick, David, 103
Rauscher, Frank J. Jr., 36–37
Reproduction of RNA Tumor Viruses, 78
Research Center for Genitourinary Tuberculosis, 52
Retroviral Testing and Quality Assurance Essentials for Laboratory Diagnosis, 8
Retroviruses
   actinomycin D inhibition of, 35
   antibiotics effect on, 42
   discovery of, 33–35
   Gallo's work on, 27

history of, 33
latent, 29
Rous' work with, 33–34
Reverse transcriptase, 35–36,
   73–74
RO318959, 103
Rous, Francis Peyton, 33–34
Rous virus, 44
Rutgers-Presbyterian Hospital
   Laboratory for the Study of
   Proliferative Diseases, 44

S
Sanger, Heinz Ludwig, 15
Saquinavir, 103
Semen, 46, 49–50
Sexual transmission
   of AIDS, 23, 49
   of tuberculosis, 52–54, 57, 62
Sezary T-cell leukemia, 29
Simian-avium mycobacteria
   group, 114, 117
Slim disease, 83–85
*Slim Disease: A New Disease in
   Uganda,* 83
"Slow viruses," 75
Syphilis, 58

T
T cells, 24–25. *See also* CD4+
   cells

Tabi, Djamel, 38
Teas, Jane, 28
Temin, Howard, 35–36
T-helper cells, 25
Tubercular "consumption,"
   83–84, 87
Tubercular mycobacteria, 109–110
Tuberculosis. *See also* Fowl
   tuberculosis
   as AIDS-defining illnesses,
      8, 105
   Alexander-Jackson's work
      with, 71
   antiretrovirals effect on, 6
   in cats, 29
   CD4 counts affected by, 90,
      93
   country-specific prevalence
      of, 82
   drug-resistant, 116
   highly active antiretrovi-
      ral therapy effects on,
      104–105
   HIV and, 8, 111, 114
   lymph node involvement by,
      14, 30
   macrophage destruction by,
      96–97
   microscopic image of, 14
   mortality caused by, 12, 83
   multidrug-resistant, 117

neck lymphadenopathy
  caused by, 13
as opportunistic infection, 86
penile ulcer caused by, 56, 58
prevalence of, 82–83
prostatic, 52–53
sexual transmission of, 52–54, 57, 62
in swine, 66
in twentieth-century, 83
vulvar, 55
wasting syndrome versus, 83
Tuberculosis epididymitis, 52

U
Ultraviolet Spectrogramic Microscope Studies of Rous Sarcoma Virus Cultured in Cell Free Medium, 44
University of Maryland, 9

V
Viral load, 102
Viral load test, 102
Visna, 75
Vulvar tuberculosis, 55

W
Wasting syndrome, 83, 85, 87, 115
Western blots, 9–10
World Health Organization, 8

Z
Zworykin, Vladimir, 108

www.ingramcontent.com/pod-product-compliance
Lightning Source LLC
Chambersburg PA
CBHW051808170526
45167CB00005B/1929